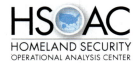
HOMELAND SECURITY
OPERATIONAL ANALYSIS CENTER

Characterization of the Synthetic Opioid Threat Profile to Inform Inspection and Detection Solutions

BRYCE PARDO, LOIS M. DAVIS, MELINDA MOORE

Published in 2019

This work is dedicated to the memory of our friend and colleague
Melinda Moore
1950–2019

Preface

The U.S. Department of Homeland Security (DHS) asked the Homeland Security Operational Analysis Center (HSOAC) to undertake an independent assessment and analysis of the synthetic opioid problem to help identify and inform inspection and detection process options. Specifically, DHS asked us to complete the following four tasks:

1. Explore available law enforcement data to evaluate general trends in seizures and the chemical profile evolution of the supply of synthetic opioids.
2. Identify national overdose trends, based on analyses of available data.
3. Characterize the delivery mechanisms used to transport, traffic, and distribute synthetic opioids, based on data from seizures and other data sources (e.g., supplemental web scrapes and unsealed federal indictments).[1]
4. Assess chemical compounds associated with cutting and packaging synthetic opioids for retail, based on supplemental data collected.

These findings should be of interest to agencies tasked with interdicting synthetic opioids at U.S. ports of entry and the general public interested in learning more about the illicit supply of synthetic opioids. We focus most of our report and its findings for decisionmakers overseeing drug interdiction operations, particularly those at or near international mail and express consignment courier facilities.

This research was sponsored by the DHS Science and Technology Directorate and conducted within the Acquisition and Development Program of the HSOAC federally funded research and development center (FFRDC).

About the Homeland Security Operational Analysis Center

The Homeland Security Act of 2002 (Section 305 of Public Law 107-296, as codified at 6 U.S.C. § 185), authorizes the Secretary of Homeland Security, acting through the Under Secretary for Science and Technology, to establish one or more FFRDCs to provide independent analysis of homeland security issues. The RAND Corporation operates HSOAC as an FFRDC for DHS under contract HSHQDC-16-D-00007.

The HSOAC FFRDC provides the government with independent and objective analyses and advice in core areas important to the department in support of policy development, decision-

---

[1] Web scraping is a common practice that uses automation to extract data from a website, allowing text-based data to be cleaned and analyzed.

making, alternative approaches, and new ideas on issues of significance. The HSOAC FFRDC also works with and supports other federal, state, local, tribal, and public- and private-sector organizations that make up the homeland security enterprise. The HSOAC FFRDC's research is undertaken by mutual consent with DHS and is organized as a set of discrete tasks. This report presents the results of research and analysis conducted under 70RSAT18FR0000077, "Characterization of the Synthetic Opioid Threat Profile to Inform Inspection and Detection Solutions."

The results presented in this report do not necessarily reflect official DHS opinion or policy.

For more information on HSOAC, see www.rand.org/hsoac. For more information on this publication, see www.rand.org/t/RR2969.

Contents

Figures and Tables

Figures

Tables

Summary

According to the National Center for Health Statistics, the percentage of drug overdose deaths involving synthetic opioids other than methadone increased, on average, by 18 percent each year between 1999 and 2006; although there was no change between 2006 and 2013, the rate dramatically increased by 88 percent per year between 2013 and 2016. By 2016, synthetic opioids had become the leading cause of U.S. drug overdose deaths, surpassing those involving heroin or semisynthetic opioids (e.g., hydrocodone or oxycodone) (Hedegaard, Warner, and Miniño, 2017). In 16 states, the overdose death rates from synthetic opioids at least doubled between 2015 to 2017, with West Virginia, Ohio, and New Hampshire having the highest death rates from synthetic opioids. Although several synthetic opioids have legitimate medical applications, most of these overdoses are due to illicitly manufactured synthetic opioids, which are often used as adulterants in heroin or pressed into counterfeit prescription tablets (Gladden, Martinez, and Seth, 2016; Ciccarone, 2017).

According to law enforcement in North America and Europe, illicitly produced synthetic opioids, such as fentanyl, are imported—with China indicated as the primary source—and arrive at international mail facilities and express consignment carriers. Additionally, some portion of illicit fentanyl arrives smuggled over the borders from Mexico and Canada. Challenges in detecting and targeting fentanyl and other synthetic opioids include the sheer volume of packages and vehicles that arrive at ports of entry (POEs), the fact that the substances are usually transferred in small amounts to avoid detection, and the rapid evolution of distribution networks, with online vendors appearing to be warehousing synthetic opioids in the United States and supplying substances through the domestic U.S. Postal Service (USPS). Holding inventory in the United States poses a substantial challenge to frontline interdiction efforts because items shipped within the domestic postal system are the jurisdiction of the USPS Inspection Service, not U.S. Customs and Border Protection (CBP).

The U.S. Department of Homeland Security asked the Homeland Security Operational Analysis Center to undertake an independent assessment and analysis of the synthetic opioid problem to help identify and inform inspection and detection process options and to aid with the development of capability requirements to improve the inspection process. Specifically, the department asked us to complete the following four tasks:

1. Characterize national-, state-, and county-level overdose trends.
2. Descriptively assess trends in synthetic opioid supply over time across regions.

3. Characterize the delivery mechanisms used to transport, traffic, and distribute synthetic opioids.
4. Assess chemical compounds associated with adulterating and packaging synthetic opioids for retail, based on supplemental data collected.

To address these four tasks, we used a multimethod approach to review and analyze data and information from a variety of sources. These included congressional reports and testimonies, publicly available data from the U.S. Drug Enforcement Administration's (DEA's) National Forensic Laboratory Information System (NFLIS) and from CBP, seizure data from public reports and congressional testimony, drug overdose mortality data from the Centers for Disease Control and Prevention, unsealed U.S. Department of Justice indictments, and information from surface-web vendors' websites and internet drug forums.[2]

Key Findings

There Has Been an Upward Trend in Synthetic Opioid Overdose Deaths over Time

Data for 2015 through 2017 indicate that synthetic opioid deaths are on the rise and reaching exceedingly high levels in some states and especially in some counties. In 2017, the ten states with the highest unadjusted per capita drug overdose death rates involving synthetic opioids were, in descending order of rate, West Virginia, Ohio, New Hampshire, Maryland, Massachusetts, Maine, Connecticut, Rhode Island, Delaware, and Kentucky. Understanding the levels and trends of these mortality data reflects only the tip of the iceberg, given that not all overdose fatalities are accurately recorded and the large number of nonfatal drug overdoses on top of those that result in death.

Nonetheless, these data can be used to help CBP (as well as the USPS Inspection Service) target inbound packages from abroad that are destined for markets where synthetic opioids pose the greatest threat. Refocusing additional detection resources on parcels destined for areas of high mortality might improve interdiction efforts. Although overdose death data might not be a perfect proxy for where incoming packages are addressed, county hot spots and associated ZIP Codes could be a first-level proxy for destinations of imported drug shipments.

Seizures of Synthetic Opioids Have Been Increasing over Time, and Markets Are Evolving

Using publicly available data, our analyses indicate that seizures containing fentanyl and other related substances have been increasing over time. In addition, the growing variation of fentanyl analogs reported to NFLIS suggests market evolution. Looking at these data across the United States, we see variation in the supply of synthetic opioids, such as fentanyl. Several regions report high per capita rates of seizures that contain fentanyl and other related chemicals. The New England census region (Connecticut, Maine, Massachusetts, New Hampshire, Rhode Island, and Vermont) and East North Central census region (including parts of Appalachia) report the highest per capita rates. The upward trend in NFLIS reports is positively correlated with overdose death rates for synthetic opioids. Without a doubt, the supply of these substances to domestic drug markets is increasing the harms that drug users experience.

---

[2]   The surface web is that portion of the World Wide Web that is readily available to the general public and searchable with standard web search engines.

There is also considerable geographic variation in the types of chemicals present. In states in New England, fentanyl predominates in NFLIS observations. In contrast, data for such states as Ohio and some in the Middle Atlantic show greater variation in the types of chemicals reported. Assuming that testing protocols and referent libraries do not vary much across laboratories that report to NFLIS, this variation suggests that these markets might be supplied by different sources. States that lack variation might have fewer suppliers or entrants to the market and might be supplied by more-traditional drug trafficking organizations, while states that report greater variation in seizure data might be supplied by online vendors from China, which offer a multitude of ever-changing analogs. Drug law enforcement efforts should be tailored to these different sources of supply.

DEA data from NFLIS indicate that about 70 percent of seizures containing fentanyl are fentanyl only (i.e., contain no other drug). Only about one-quarter of fentanyl-related seizures in NFLIS contain heroin. Without knowing whether seizures are of product at the wholesale level or retail level, we cannot determine from NFLIS where in the supply chain the mixing is occurring. In addition, assessing illicit market activity based on public data provides only a rough insight into the evolution of the supply of illicit synthetic opioids.

Our analysis of public NFLIS data at the state level suggests variation in supply sources, with fentanyl analogs concentrated in some states, but not in others. Understanding the variation on the ground in these different sources of supply could help improve law enforcement's response. If certain regions are supplied largely by online vendors—as indicated by the proportion of analogs reported in a state—law enforcement might want to redirect detection resources to focus on inbound parcels destined to certain areas. In markets supplied by more-traditional trafficking organizations, law enforcement will need to prioritize traditional investigation and disruption techniques to target and dismantle transnational trafficking and distribution networks.

Another finding from this research is the lack of understanding of drug seizures that contain heroin, cocaine, or methamphetamine mixed with synthetic opioids, such as fentanyl. Overdose deaths from these other classes of drugs show a growing share that include synthetic opioids (Pardo and Reuter, 2018). DEA data reported in NFLIS and analyzed for our study suggest that about one-quarter of fentanyl seizures also contain heroin, with minor shares containing cocaine or other drugs. However, it is unclear where drug mixing is taking place (at wholesale or closer to retail markets).

In addition, the manufacture, importation, and distribution of counterfeit pills and tablets containing fentanyl and other synthetic opioids present unique challenges to public health and safety. These processes combine a traditional drug supply issue with one of trademark infringement. Drug users consuming these items might be at greater risk of overdose because they might be under the impression that they are using pharmaceutical-grade products of known purity and consistency. Unlike with powders, which are known to vary in quality and purity from bag to bag, those consuming pills might not consider that such tablets could contain an unknown amount of potent synthetic opioids. This is further complicated by the fact that some counterfeit tablets are made to resemble benzodiazepines rather than prescription opioids (DEA, 2018c). Data collection and analysis systems do not readily allow us to fully quantify the harm that counterfeit tablets pose, which could be greater than that of powdered fentanyl, given that these items add layers of misinformation that conceal overdose risk. Further, the counterfeit pill phenomenon could lead to greater exposure to fentanyl and related substances because pills generally appeal to non–injection drug–using populations, whose opioid tolerance might be lower.

Methods of Trafficking Synthetic Opioids Vary

The production of highly potent synthetic opioids introduces considerable challenges to drug interdiction. Unlike traditional drugs, synthetic opioids can be produced anywhere by anyone with knowledge of basic synthetic chemistry and access to chemicals; their potency-to-weight ratio makes them profitable enough to ship tens of grams via the international postal system or conceal small amounts in vehicles, other conveyance methods, or hidden with legitimate commerce. Inexpensive shipping and the rise of e-commerce allow just about anyone to acquire these substances from the comfort of one's own home. Between 2013 and 2017, the volume of international packages inbound to the United States has almost quintupled. In 2017, USPS handled nearly 500 million packages that arrived in the United States from abroad (Permanent Subcommittee on Investigations, 2018), presenting a daunting challenge to screening and detection efforts.

Law enforcement reports and seizure data suggest that synthetic opioids arrive in the United States not only by mail or express consignment carriers but also via traditional drug trafficking routes across the southwest border. Mexican and Dominican drug trafficking organizations have been implicated in the importation of fentanyl, often smuggled over the border.[3] Fewer data are available for understanding traditional smuggling routes for fentanyl. Smuggling methods for synthetic opioids across the southwest border appear to be the same for those used for traditional drug threats, such as cocaine, heroin, and methamphetamine. These include concealment in compartments in vehicles, as well as hidden on persons. Law enforcement reports suggest that fentanyl seized at land POEs at the southwest border is of lower purity, often in powders and sometimes in pressed counterfeit tablet formulations. Absent chemical analysis of these seizures, it is hard to ascertain why these seizures, even large multi-kilogram seizures, contain low amounts of fentanyl.

The more novel method for supply of fentanyl is via online vendors that mail product directly to buyers. Analysis based on publicly available data provides insights into some of the mechanisms that online vendors use. Many online vendors analyzed claim to employ methods to circumvent customs. The supply chain of fentanyl and synthetic opioids arriving by air is not always the same as those for heroin and cocaine. First, vendors regularly use the postal or other private consignment couriers to transmit packages to customers, generally shipping orders no larger than 1 kg. Larger amounts are offered upon request, but those might originate from domestic warehouses near customers.

Second, the discussion by many online vendors of warehousing product in Europe, the United States, and elsewhere to avoid detection suggests that suppliers understand risk and take steps to reduce it. At this time, there is no way to know what share of inventory is warehoused outside China. However, knowing that inventory arrives in the United States through bulk container and cargo shipments might necessitate a recalibration of law enforcement strategy to focus on cargo shipments from countries known to produce synthetic opioids, such as China.

Third, vendors appear to understand customs and detection risks, preferring to ship through the international postal system, such as USPS or Express Mail Service. Vendors men-

---

[3] In this report, *Dominican* is a descriptor for something from the Dominican Republic, not the Commonwealth of Dominica.

tion that the risk of interdiction is low, and many offer to reship orders at no cost should packages be lost, stolen, or interdicted.

But more to the point is that, if vendors are to be believed and their rate of success in shipping product to buyers in the United States is almost always successful, customs is perhaps seizing only a small proportion of total shipments. Alternatively, online vendors face little risk of arrest, let alone prosecution, so their reported rates of success could be a marketing scheme because they can likely tolerate loss. Given that the supply of these substances is unconventional, with vendors openly discussing their product and exclusive use of the postal system, law enforcement should start to think more creatively—if it has not done so already—to obtain additional information about packages. Such efforts could include initiating more controlled buys with the goal of informing detection metrics.

Additional Information Is Needed on the Chemicals Associated with Cutting and Packaging of Synthetic Opioids for Retail

Our analysis of online vendors and marketplace listings suggests that most of the product on offer from retailers overseas is highly pure, which coincides with CBP seizure analyses described in law enforcement reports. A review of online vendors' product descriptions indicates that most items sold in the marketplace are of powder formulation. This finding supports law enforcement reports that high-purity product in powder form is seized in mail facilities. According to DEA seizure analyses, the share of fentanyl found in individual counterfeit tablets is relatively small (approximately 1.5 mg of a counterfeit tablet that might weigh as little as 120 mg), suggesting that the rest of the tablet contains some other diluent or adulterant.

According to DEA reports of NFLIS data, two-thirds of analyzed fentanyl cases contain no other drug mixtures. However, about one-quarter of fentanyl seizures between 2014 and 2016 also contained heroin, followed by other opioids, at 4 percent. This and the fact that fentanyl is often offered as heroin or as a prescription opioid are notable insights. Analysis of heroin seizures in recent years could provide further understanding into cutting agents used in the retail sale of fentanyl products. If dealers in the United States are replacing heroin with fentanyl to reduce costs, they might be using the same or similar bulking and cutting agents.

However, without assessing individual seizure data, we are limited in our ability to understand the cutting and bulking agents included in retail distribution of fentanyl and novel synthetic opioids. Analyses of recent fentanyl seizures conducted by DEA show that the most-common cutting agents are lactose and mannitol. However, these seizure analyses are not representative, and reasons that seizures at land POEs (i.e., smuggled from Mexico) are of such low purity and the extent to which fentanyl is mixed with other drugs are unclear.

Any of several hypotheses, some of which are not mutually exclusive, could explain the low purity of fentanyl arriving from Mexico. Seizures of tablets might contain mostly diluents to mimic the weight of common prescription medications. Powder seizures might be mixed with diluents or other drugs, such as heroin or cocaine—although available seizure data do not allow us to determine this conclusively. Alternatively, the low purity of seized fentanyl might be due to poor synthesis and purification methods that leave other impurities and reagents behind. At this time, we lack the available data to make strong claims.

Recommendations

The findings from our analysis suggest a series of recommendations; we list them here but develop them in more detail in Chapter Six:

- Use mortality or other poisoning and injury data to inform the targeting of packages from abroad.
- Improve data collection and analysis of drug seizures by standardizing measures collected across all international mail facilities, express consignment carriers, and land POEs.
- Enhance cooperation with other federal agencies and departments to better understand the nature and supply of synthetic opioids.
- Enhance collaboration and exchange data with counterparts in law enforcement and border protection in other countries.
- Conduct controlled deliveries for analytic purposes.
- Consider targeting bulk shipments hidden in cargo from China at POEs.

Acknowledgments

We would like to acknowledge the staff of the U.S. Department of Homeland Security's Science and Technology Directorate (S&T) and U.S. Customs and Border Protection for their thoughtful input into this study and for providing access to staff, as well as to data and other information needed to inform our analyses. These individuals include

- Rosanna Robertson, program manager, Office of Mission and Capability Support, S&T
- Shannon Fox, Office of National Laboratories, Chemical Security Analysis Center, S&T
- Keith Bayha, Office of Mission Capability Support, S&T
- Candice Williams, Chemical and Biological Defense Program, S&T
- Eric Levine, Office of National Laboratories, Chemical Security Analysis Center, S&T
- Steve Weiss, U.S. Customs and Border Protection.

We also wish to thank Isaac Porche, director of the Homeland Security Operational Analysis Center's Acquisition and Development Program, for his guidance throughout this project. We also acknowledge the project administrative support of Hunter Granger and Daniel Spagiare.

Shawn Smith and Alice Kim provided research support to key components of the study. We thank them for their input and excellent support.

Lastly, we appreciate the thoughtful insights provided by our technical reviewers, Beau Kilmer and Jonathan P. Caulkins. Rosalie Liccardo Pacula also provided valuable feedback on our approach.

Abbreviations

AED	advance electronic data
CBP	U.S. Customs and Border Protection
CDC	Centers for Disease Control and Prevention
DEA	U.S. Drug Enforcement Administration
DHS	U.S. Department of Homeland Security
DOJ	U.S. Department of Justice
ECC	express consignment carrier
ECO	express consignment operator
EMCDDA	European Monitoring Centre for Drugs and Drug Addiction
EMS	Express Mail Service
FAQ	frequently asked question
FFRDC	federally funded research and development center
FSPP	Fentanyl Signature Profiling Program
FY	fiscal year
HHI	Herfindahl–Hirschman Index
HSOAC	Homeland Security Operational Analysis Center
ICD-10	International Statistical Classification of Diseases and Related Health Problems, tenth revision
IMF	international mail facility
NFLIS	National Forensic Laboratory Information System
NSO	novel synthetic opioid
POE	port of entry
S&T	Science and Technology Directorate
UPS	United Parcel Service

URL   uniform resource locator

USPIS   U.S. Postal Inspection Service

USPS   U.S. Postal Service

WHO   World Health Organization

CHAPTER ONE

Introduction

Since 2013, the rate of drug overdose deaths that involved synthetic opioids in the United States has grown rapidly. According to the National Center for Health Statistics, the rate of drug overdose deaths that involved synthetic opioids other than methadone increased, on average, 18 percent each year between 1999 and 2006, with no change between 2006 and 2013.[1] However, the rate then dramatically increased by 88 percent per year between 2013 and 2016. By 2016, synthetic opioids became the leading cause of drug overdose deaths in the United States, surpassing those involving heroin or semisynthetic opioids (e.g., hydrocodone or oxycodone) (Hedegaard, Warner, and Miniño, 2017). The largest increase in synthetic opioid overdose death rates was in people ages 25 to 44—specifically, men in that age range (CDC, 2018b). Rates of increase also varied geographically. In ten states, the overdose death rates from synthetic opioids at least doubled between 2015 and 2016, with New Hampshire, West Virginia, and Massachusetts having the highest death rates from synthetic opioids (CDC, 2018b).

CDC estimated that, in 2015 alone, there were 52,404 drug overdose deaths in the United States, with 33,091 (63.1 percent) involving opioids; the largest rate increases (between 2014 to 2015) were for deaths involving synthetic opioids other than methadone (72.2 percent) (Seth et al., 2018). For 2016, CDC estimated there were 63,600 drug overdose deaths, with 66 percent of those deaths being the result of opioids, including fentanyl and novel synthetic opioids (NSOs) (Hedegaard, Warner, and Miniño, 2017).

Likewise, reports of the numbers of exhibits submitted to state and local crime laboratories for fentanyl increased dramatically, from 978 in 2013 to more than 59,000 in 2017 (National Forensic Laboratory Information System [NFLIS], 2018). There are regional differences as well in the number of fentanyl-confirmed reports. For example, in 2017, of the fentanyl exhibits reported in NFLIS, three-quarters were recorded by laboratories in the Northeast (24,638 reports) and in the Midwest (18,047 reports) (NFLIS, 2018). We note that these are counts for fentanyl, not other analogs or other synthetic opioids. As we show later, the numbers involving other synthetic opioids reported in laboratories have also increased in recent years.

Illicitly produced fentanyl and NSOs arrive from abroad, with China indicated as the primary source (O'Connor, 2017). These synthetic opioids arrive in U.S. markets directly

---

[1] The term *synthetic opioids* applies to synthesized opioids that are not derived from poppy. In drug overdose death data from the Centers for Disease Control and Prevention (CDC), *synthetic opioids* includes such substances as fentanyl, fentanyl analogs, other novel synthetic opioids (e.g., U-47700), tramadol, and other synthesized opioids that might or might not be prescribed. It does not include methadone, which has a distinct International Statistical Classification of Diseases and Related Problems, tenth revision (ICD-10) code even though it is synthesized. Throughout this report, the term generally refers to illicitly manufactured fentanyl and other related novel opioids that are synthesized outside of regulated settings and are intended to be consumed by people who use drugs (Gladden, Martinez, and Seth, 2016).

from Chinese manufacturers via the post or private couriers (e.g., United Parcel Service [UPS], FedEx), smuggled from Mexico, or smuggled from Canada as pressed counterfeit prescription pills or in powder form (Baum, 2017; O'Connor, 2017). At this time, it is unknown what share of fentanyl enters by each port of entry (POE) or from what original source, although U.S. Drug Enforcement Administration (DEA) suggests that some portion of fentanyl might be produced in Mexico using precursors from China (DEA, 2017). U.S. Customs and Border Protection (CBP) has reported that, in fiscal year (FY) 2017, about 675 kg of fentanyl were seized, with 80 percent of the bulk weight of those seizures being seized at POEs (including border crossings, mail, and express consignment carrier [ECC] facilities), while the remainder was interdicted at CBP checkpoints (Owen, 2018).

Synthetic opioids are openly available for purchase on the Internet from vendors overseas that distribute these substances in packages through the postal and parcel systems. These substances arrive from abroad at U.S. POEs, such as international mail facilities (IMFs) and ECC operations facilities alongside everyday correspondence and items of general commerce. CBP has noted a substantial increase in the volume and number of seizures of packages and parcels containing fentanyl and related substances from China (Owen, 2018).

Between late 2014 and the beginning of 2017, the U.S. Postal Service (USPS) Inspection Service (USPIS) seized nearly 100 parcels that contained synthetic opioids, or an average of about 37 in a 12-month period (Baum, 2017). CBP reported that, in FY 2017 alone, it seized 227 parcels containing fentanyl, totaling 42 kg, at IMFs and 118 parcels containing fentanyl, totaling 110 kg, at ECC facilities (Owen, 2018).

There are challenges in detecting fentanyl and other synthetic opioids shipped through the international mail system and ECCs. The sheer volume of packages makes it infeasible for USPS and ECCs to inspect every package (Permanent Subcommittee on Investigations, 2018). For example, international package volume that USPS handles has almost doubled, going from 150 million packages in FY 2013 to 275 million in FY 2016. In comparison, in 2016, approximately 65.7 million packages from abroad were handled by the three major express consignment operators (ECOs) in the United States (Permanent Subcommittee on Investigations, 2018).[2] In 2017 alone, with respect to USPS's international package volume, the number of packages from overseas reached more than 498 million (Permanent Subcommittee on Investigations, 2018).

Sending small quantities of fentanyl and NSOs halfway around the world via the international postal system is economically viable. Several online vendors we examined ship as little as 10 g of fentanyl to buyers outside China. According to China Post, the cost of airmailing a parcel to the United States weighing up to 20 g is ¥6, or about $0.90.[3] Sending a 500-g parcel from China by airmail to the United States costs roughly ¥93, or $13.60. These shipment costs are a fraction of the cost of the drugs in question. The price of fentanyl sold online from vendors can range from $200 to $700 for as little as 10 g and $2,000 to $5,000 for 500 g. A search of ECO shipping rates suggests that a 1-kg parcel can be shipped from China to the United States for about $100, which makes shipping by private courier economically viable for producers in China, which often waive shipping fees for customers.

---

[2]   The three major ECOs are UPS, FedEx, and DHL Express (Permanent Subcommittee on Investigations, 2018).

[3]   See China Post, undated, for postal fees.

The preferred supply method of online vendors is Express Mail Service (EMS), a cooperative with a network that delivers letters and packages through each member country's postal operations, including USPS (Permanent Subcommittee on Investigations, 2018).[4] CBP can use advance electronic data (AED), which include such information as sender and recipient name and address and a description of the package contents provided by the shipper at the time of package drop-off, to identify suspicious packages to target for further inspection. USPS relies on foreign postal operators to collect AED on internationally shipped packages; however, the international postal community has not fully adopted it (Permanent Subcommittee on Investigations, 2018). As a result, in 2017, only 36 percent of packages sent to the United States included AED. In contrast, parcels shipped through ECCs have AED, allowing identification of suspicious packages.[5] This, along with Fourth Amendment protections against searches and seizures, is one reason online vendors claim to prefer EMS to ECCs for shipping product. In late 2018, Congress passed the Synthetics Trafficking and Overdose Prevention (STOP) Act (Pub. L. 115-271, 2018, Title VIII, Miscellaneous; Subtitle A, Synthetics Trafficking and Overdose Prevention), requiring USPS to obtain AED for all packages arriving from China. The impacts that this new statutory requirement will have on the importation of synthetic opioids by mail remain to be seen.

Although CBP operates at the nine major IMFs where international mail arrives from more than 180 countries, the lack of uniform advance cargo information to aid in targeting shipments makes it difficult to interdict fentanyl and other drugs (Perez, 2017). Furthermore, although China is the primary source of supply for fentanyl and its precursors, to obfuscate package origin and reduce the risk of seizure, online sellers sometimes divert packages (i.e., transship) through other countries before those packages arrive in the United States (Permanent Subcommittee on Investigations, 2018).

To avoid detection when supplying fentanyl and other synthetic opioids by mail, vendors usually transfer substances in small quantities. Furthermore, the distribution methods appear to be evolving. Online vendors claim to be warehousing synthetic opioids in the United States, supplying substances via USPS. According to indictments and some observations reported in CBP seizure data, synthetic opioids warehoused in the United States likely arrive in bulk through cargo shipments, often in containers labeled as holding other chemicals. Domestic warehousing circumvents CBP interdiction efforts targeting small parcels that arrive at IMFs because items shipped within the domestic postal system are the jurisdiction of USPIS.

Project Objective and Research Tasks

The U.S. Department of Homeland Security (DHS) asked the Homeland Security Operational Analysis Center (HSOAC) to undertake an independent assessment and analysis of the

---

[4]   International mail packages shipped through USPS enter the United States primarily through one of five international service centers at John F. Kennedy International Airport in New York, O'Hare International Airport in Chicago, Los Angeles International Airport, San Francisco International Airport, and Miami International Airport (Permanent Subcommittee on Investigations, 2018).

[5]   In the Trade Act of 2002 (Pub. L. 107-210), Congress required that, for security purposes following the September 11, 2001, terrorist attacks, ECOs collect certain information on all packages shipped through their networks. Thus, all packages shipped by ECOs have AED (Permanent Subcommittee on Investigations, 2018).

synthetic opioid problem to help identify and inform inspection and detection process options and to inform the development of capability requirements to improve the inspection process.

Specifically, DHS asked us to complete the following four tasks:

1. Explore available law enforcement data to evaluate general trends in seizures and the chemical profile evolution of the supply of synthetic opioids.
2. Identify national overdose trends based on analyses of available data.
3. Characterize the delivery mechanisms used to transport/traffic/distribute synthetic opioids based on data from seizures and other data sources (e.g., supplemental web-scrapes and unsealed federal indictments).
4. Assess chemical compounds associated with cutting/packaging synthetic opioids for retail from supplemental data collection.

As discussed in the next section, our findings in this report rely on publicly available data sources. We have supplemented our data analyses with primary data collection efforts to provide some additional dimensions of the problem.

Methods

To address the four tasks listed in the technical execution plan, we used a multimethod approach to review and analyze data and information from a variety of sources (see Table 1.1), including congressional reports and testimonies, publicly available data from DEA's NFLIS, CBP POE seizure data provided by S&T, seizure data from public reports and congressional testimony, CDC overdose mortality data, unsealed U.S. Department of Justice (DOJ) indictments, and information from surface-web vendors' websites.

Table 1.1
Data Sources, by Task

Data Source			Task			
Source	Database or Report	Type	Task 1	Task 2	Task 3	Task 4
CDC	Multiple Cause of Death Data[a]	Death certificates		x		
S&T	POE seizure data	Individual seizure events	x		x	
DEA	Public NFLIS reports	Drug seizure counts	x			
DEA	Unclassified FSPP data	Fentanyl seizure analyses				x
HSOAC	Surface-web vendors	Online retail sale data	x		x	
HSOAC	Peer-reviewed literature	Descriptive data on adulterants				x
DOJ, Congress, and federal agencies	Public reports, indictments, testimonies	Descriptive data on suppliers and trafficking of synthetic opioids	x		x	x

NOTE: S&T = Science and Technology Directorate. FSPP = Fentanyl Signature Profiling Program.
[a] CDC, 2018a.

Specifically, for task 1, we analyzed publicly available NFLIS data to descriptively assess trends in seizures of synthetic opioids over time across regions. For task 2, we analyzed national-, state-, and county-level drug overdose death data from CDC's National Vital Statistics System (available for the period through 2017) to characterize synthetic opioid overdose trends at the national, state, and county levels. We also mapped "high-risk" counties and cities with their corresponding ZIP Codes to inform S&T's and CBP's understanding of where synthetic opioids might be destined given overdose deaths as proxy for consumption. For task 3, we conducted web scrapes of three surface-web online marketplaces from Asia (Exporters India, Mfrbee, and Tradett), reviewed unsealed DOJ indictments of Chinese vendors, and conducted in-depth analyses of several surface-web vendors that appear most frequently in search engine results.[6] For task 4, we examined drug mixtures from NFLIS reported by DEA and analyzed qualitative information on packaging and transport from unsealed DOJ federal indictments of Chinese vendors, federal law enforcement reports, analysis of popular vendors, and web scrapes.

Overall, our analyses for tasks 1, 3, and 4 presented here are based on publicly available data. We would have liked to explore additional drug seizure data from DEA to evaluate general trends in chemical profile evolution, mixtures with other substances, purity, and location. Instead, our analyses presented here are based on publicly available seizure totals from annual reports, unclassified law enforcement reports, and congressional testimony. For task 4, we have relied on unclassified drug signature profiling reports.

In each of the following chapters, we provide additional detail on the data sources and methods used for each task. We note in the relevant chapters the limitations of such data sources and, in Chapter Six, discuss what additional data might be informative to address key research and policy questions.

Road Map for This Report

Chapter Two (addressing task 2) provides the overall policy context to understand the magnitude of the synthetic opioid problem by first presenting national overdose trends and then examining state and county data that might indicate areas of high consumption of synthetic opioids. The chapter first presents data at the state level, followed by data for counties with the highest rates of overdose deaths. We then provide more-granular targeting data by mapping ZIP Codes to a list of high-risk counties and cities (defined as those that have double the national rate of synthetic opioid overdose deaths) to inform S&T's and CBP's understanding of high-use markets for synthetic opioids.

Chapter Three (addressing task 1) utilizes law enforcement seizure data submitted to NFLIS to examine national and regional trends in seizures of fentanyl and NSOs and the evolution of chemical trends over time and across regions.

Chapter Four (addressing task 3) draws on data from web scrapes of three surface-web online marketplaces,[7] an exhaustive comparative analysis of eight popular online vendors, and

---

[6] Web scraping is a common practice that uses automation to extract data from a website, allowing text-based data to be cleaned and analyzed.

[7] The surface web is that portion of the World Wide Web that is readily available to the general public and searchable with standard web search engines.

a review of unsealed DOJ indictments of Chinese vendors to characterize the delivery mechanisms used to transport, traffic, and distribute synthetic opioids. In the law enforcement–sensitive version of this report, this chapter also includes findings from our analysis of privileged seizure data.

To assess chemical compounds associated with cutting and packaging synthetic opioids for retail, Chapter Five (addressing task 4) draws on information from a variety of sources, including unsealed DOJ indictments of Chinese vendors, federal law enforcement reports, our analysis of popular vendors, and web scrapes. Findings in this chapter also come from peer-reviewed articles and unclassified DEA chemical signature reports.

Chapter Six summarizes our key conclusions for each of the four tasks and offers recommendations to DHS and CBP, which might inform their drug interdiction strategies.

CHAPTER TWO

Emerging Trends in Fatal Synthetic Opioid Overdoses

Drug overdose deaths have been on the rise in the United States during the past two decades, driven mainly by opioids. Figure 2.1 shows the drug overdose death rates for the United States by year and drug class. Multiple Cause of Death Data show that, beginning in 2013, rates of overdose deaths due to synthetic opioids have increased dramatically over time. Between 2013 and 2017, the synthetic opioid overdose death rate jumped from one per 100,000 population to nine per 100,000 population, far surpassing the 2017 death rates due to heroin (4.9 per 100,000 population) or due to prescription opioids (4.4 per 100,000 population). Although the drug overdose death rate due to prescription opioids was higher than other cause categories between 2005 and 2014, by 2015, overdose deaths from heroin and synthetic opioids surpassed those due to prescription opioids. Figure 2.1 shows the steady increase in overdose death rates due to heroin since about 2010, plateauing in 2015, and synthetic opioids since about 2013.

However, Figure 2.1 obscures the diffusion of synthetic opioids across other drug classes. Simply, drug overdose deaths are not exclusive; someone who overdoses from heroin adulter-

Figure 2.1
U.S. Drug Overdose Death Rates per 100,000 Population, by Year and Drug Category

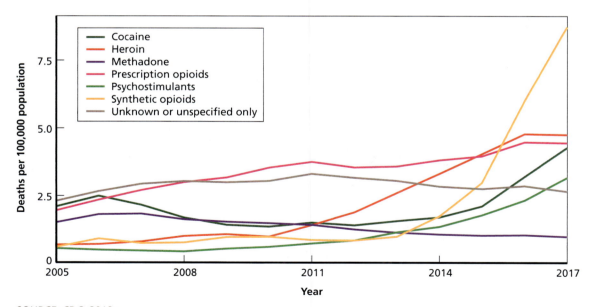

SOURCE: CDC, 2018a.
NOTE: Rates are not age-adjusted. *Psychostimulant* refers to a non-cocaine stimulant, amphetamine, or methamphetamine. Psychostimulant overdoses are largely due to methamphetamine.

ated with fentanyl will be counted as a heroin overdose and as a synthetic opioid overdose. To better illustrate this issue, Figure 2.2 shows the U.S. drug overdose death count between 2005 and 2017, separating out the share of drug overdose deaths in which a synthetic opioid was present in death certificate records. Figure 2.2 also shows the number of overdose deaths due to synthetic opioids alone (to avoid double counting, we have excluded deaths that also mention cocaine, heroin, prescription opioids, or psychostimulants). Beginning in 2014, the number of overdose deaths—across all drug death categories—that included synthetic opioids began to climb, with steep increases seen in 2016 and 2017. In 2017, 28,466 overdose death certificates mentioned synthetic opioids.

We also see a growing trend in the presence of synthetic opioids in other drug overdose cases (Figure 2.2). For heroin, starting in 2013, it appears that dealers began mixing synthetic opioids into the heroin supply and that this has increased over time. By 2017, more than half of the 15,000 heroin overdose deaths in the United States included synthetic opioids. We see a similar trend for cocaine. Starting in 2014, death records show an increase in the number of cocaine overdose death cases that also included synthetic opioids; by 2017, just over half of cases also included synthetic opioids.[1] Furthermore, Figure 2.2 indicates that users of psychostimulants (generally methamphetamine) were coming increasingly into contact with synthetic opioids.

Figure 2.2
U.S. Drug Overdose Death Count, by Year and Drug Category

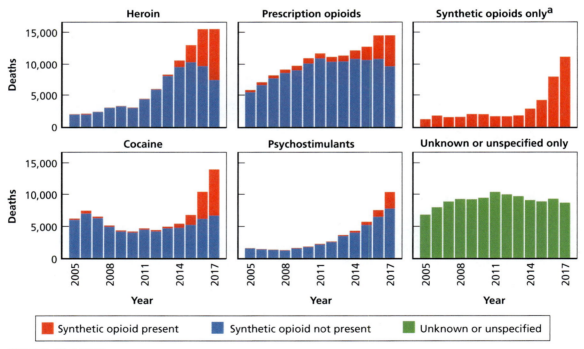

SOURCE: CDC, 2018a.
[a] Excludes cocaine, heroin, prescription opioid, and psychostimulant deaths from synthetic opioids.

---

[1]   There is less certainty surrounding where the mixing of cocaine or psychostimulants with synthetic opioids occurs. Although we suspect that dealers began switching from heroin to heroin adulterated with fentanyl (or to fentanyl by itself), given that the two are substitute opioids, drug policy researchers are still examining the stimulant-plus-fentanyl overdose

This chapter summarizes data and trends for drug overdose deaths, focusing on synthetic opioids, which, according to federal law enforcement, are illicitly imported through the mail and private courier systems, as well as smuggled over the border by drug traffickers (DEA, 2018c). The recent growth in synthetic opioid overdose deaths is driven by these illicit sources (Gladden, Martinez, and Seth, 2016). The purpose is to understand emerging national, state, and local trends, which should, in turn, help inform CBP strategies to target suspected packages destined for domestic drug markets, especially markets in which high rates of synthetic opioid deaths are occurring.

Given that fentanyl and other synthetic opioids are imported via the mail, analyzing drug mortality and morbidity indicators will be important for early warning and can help inform targeting strategies regarding inbound packages. Overdose death data do not allow us to infer the source of supply of synthetic opioids—merely where the deaths are occurring. As we discuss in Chapter Three, some markets affected by synthetic opioids might be supplied in part by transnational drug trafficking organizations rather than by producers that ship product through the mail. Therefore, examining drug overdose data alongside supply-side indicators can help to better inform law enforcement.

The approach here requires an understanding of recent trends at the most local level available. Under a data-use agreement with CDC, HSOAC researchers have analyzed individual death certificate records indicating decedents' counties of residence.

The chapter first presents data at the state level, followed by data for counties with the highest rates of synthetic opioid deaths. Per our data-use agreement with CDC, we have suppressed from publication those jurisdictions and years with fewer than ten deaths. A more granular targeting analysis would map deaths to the ZIP Code level to inform law enforcement's targeting efforts. For example, knowing the ZIP Codes associated with high use of synthetic opioids (as proxied by fatal overdoses) could provide additional targeting information to law enforcement screening incoming packages. Such additional targeting data could be helpful for canine detection units.

It should be noted that the ZIP Code targeting data can be better informed by cross-referencing them with supply-side indicators (discussed in greater detail in Chapter Three) to narrow the focus on markets likely supplied by synthetic opioids that arrive by mail and ECCs.

Methods

Mortality data are more readily available than nonfatal drug overdose data, so the HSOAC team drew from CDC's National Vital Statistics System data for 2005 through 2017. These data are provided to RAND under a data-use agreement with CDC and contain individual death certificate records on decedents' counties of residence and information on relevant ICD-10 codes for drug-involved poisonings. In early January 2019, we obtained death record data for 2016 and 2017 to complete our initial analysis presented to S&T in late 2018. The team extracted overdose death classifications by drug poisoning to examine state and county

---

death phenomenon. It might be due to dealers mixing drugs, such as cocaine and fentanyl, or users consuming both at once (known as *speedballing*).

trends.[2] We looked at both death rates and rates of change because both are important for identifying areas currently or potentially at highest risk.

Before examining the findings, we note that overdose death analysis has its limitations. Overdoses might not be tied geographically to the supply of fentanyl and NSOs. For example, a drug user might die in one location having used fentanyl that arrived by mail in a neighboring jurisdiction that has low overdose death rates. In other cases, markets might be supplied by Mexican drug trafficking organizations, which are likely to utilize traditional smuggling methods to import and distribute synthetic opioids. Therefore, the hot spots of drug overdose deaths should be thought of as approximating potential destinations of synthetic opioids.

For county-level visualizations, we have suppressed death counts for counties with fewer than 20, given that death rates based on small counts are considered unreliable (Xu et al., 2018). Because of this and other data reliability issues with drug-specific overdose deaths, all county-level visualizations display all overdose deaths. Analysis of deaths involving synthetic opioids (either alone or in combination with other drugs) are aggregated up to the state. Given the potential measurement error in drug death reporting, we have restricted our state-level visualizations to states that, according to CDC (Scholl et al., 2019), have "very good to excellent" overdose reporting in recent years, which includes Ohio, West Virginia, and states in New England.

Findings

State- and County-Level Trends

Figure 2.3 shows the per capita synthetic opioid overdose death rates, by state, for 2014 and 2017. As per our data-use agreement with CDC, we have removed states with fewer than ten deaths and those that do not have good to excellent overdose death reporting in that year. At first glance, we note an east–west divide in reported synthetic opioid overdose deaths. Here, states east of the Mississippi River reported higher rates of overdoses involving synthetic opioids. The most-recent data from CDC indicate that overdose deaths are regionally concentrated in the eastern half of the United States, with parts of Appalachia and New England most affected. The ten states with the highest rates in 2017 are, in descending order of rate, West Virginia, Ohio, New Hampshire, Maryland, Massachusetts, Maine, Connecticut, Rhode Island, Delaware, and Kentucky.

---

[2]   Drug-poisoning (overdose) deaths are identified using underlying-cause-of-death codes X40–X44, X60–X64, X85, and Y10–Y14.
   Among deaths with drug poisoning as the underlying cause, the following multiple-cause-of-death codes indicate the drug types involved: any opioid, T40.0–T40.4 and T40.6; heroin, T40.1; natural and semisynthetic opioids (prescription opioids generally fall into the latter category), T40.2; methadone, T40.3; synthetic opioids other than methadone, T40.4; cocaine, T40.5; and unknown or unspecified, T50.9.

Figure 2.3
Synthetic Opioid Overdose Death Rate per 100,000, by State, 2014 and 2017

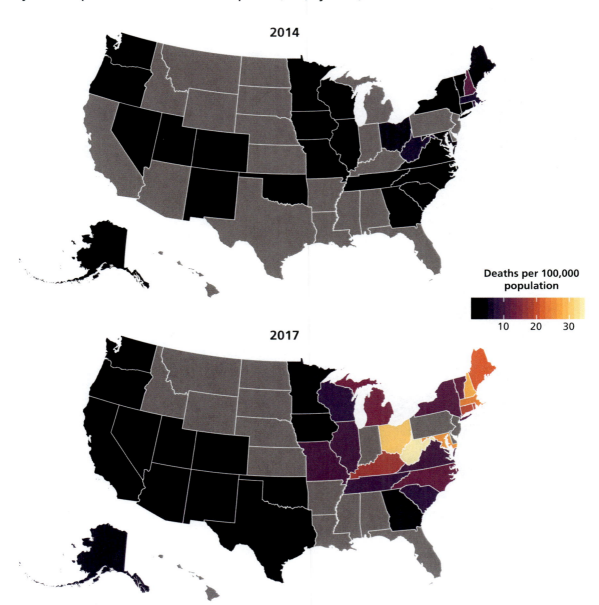

SOURCE: CDC, 2018a.
NOTE: Gray indicates a state that, according to CDC, has only fair overdose reporting and for which the data have therefore been suppressed.

In addition, within states, the highest rates of overdose death due to synthetic opioids tend to be concentrated in certain counties. For example, southern Ohio and West Virginia counties reported much higher rates of overdoses than those in the rest of the state. Figures 2.4 and 2.5 show county death rates for these hot-spot areas in Appalachia and New England for 2014 and 2017.

Figure 2.4
All-Drug Overdose Death Rate per 100,000, by County, in Ohio and West Virginia, 2014 to 2017

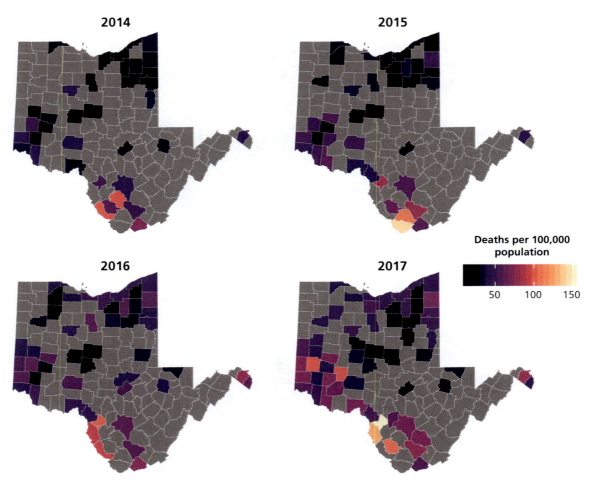

SOURCE: CDC, 2018a.
NOTE: Gray indicates a jurisdiction with fewer than 20 deaths and for which we have therefore excluded the data.

Figure 2.5
All-Overdose Death Rate per 100,000, by County, in New England, 2014 to 2017

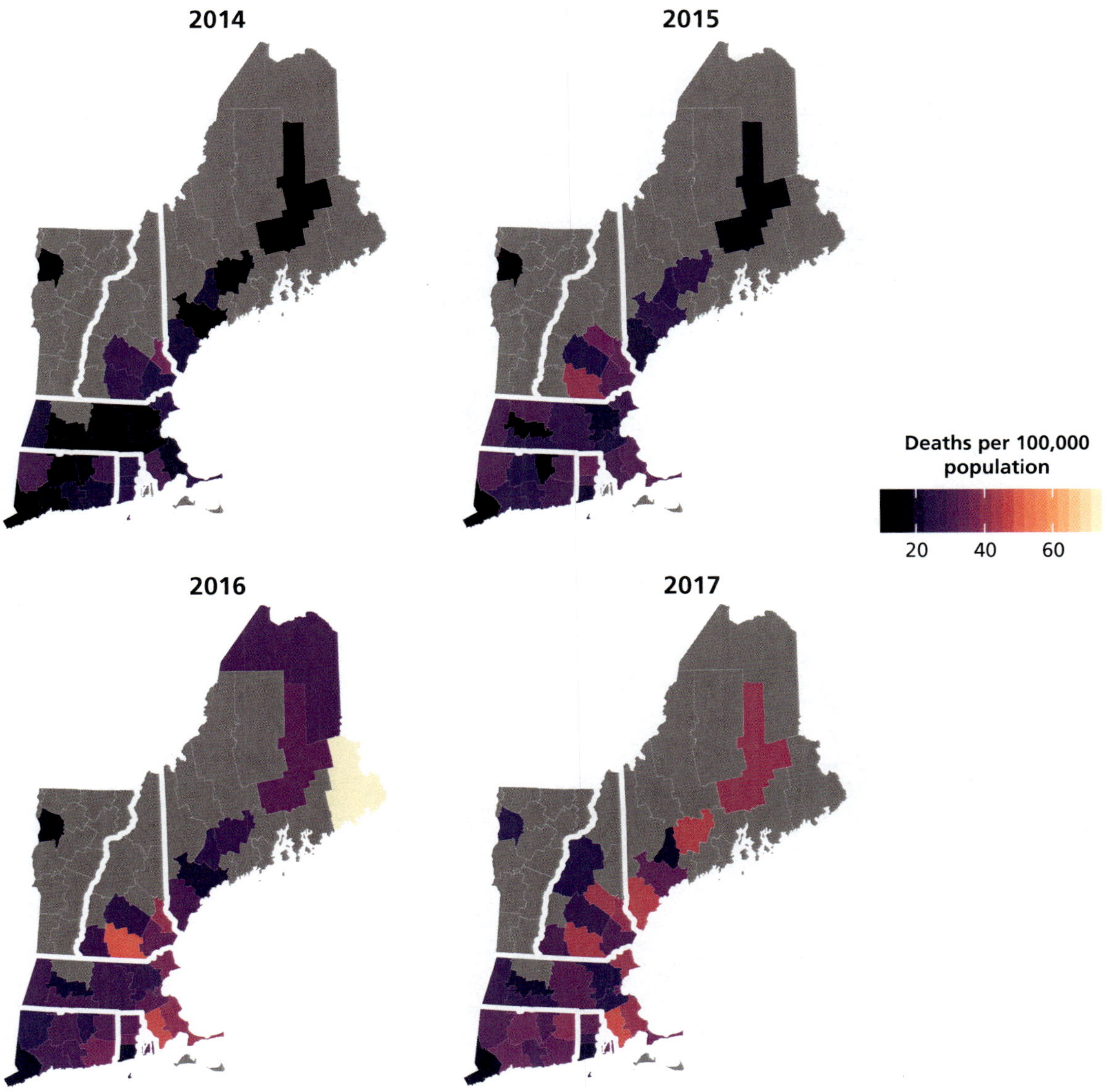

SOURCE: CDC, 2018a.
NOTE: Gray indicates a jurisdiction with fewer than 20 deaths and for which we have therefore excluded the data.

Figure 2.6 shows the increase over time at the state level in the percentage of overdoses due to heroin that contained synthetic opioids between 2014 and 2017. Here, the color coding on the maps indicates variation at the state level, with black indicating states with lower percentages of heroin overdoses that included synthetic opioids and the red to orange colors indicating states with higher percentages of such overdoses. In 2014, the highest percentage of heroin overdoses that included synthetic opioids was 60 percent; but, by 2017, the highest percentage of heroin overdoses that included synthetic opioids topped out at 80 percent in some states. The maps show a dramatic increase between 2014 and 2017 in the percentage of heroin

Figure 2.6
Percentage of Heroin Overdose Deaths That Included Synthetic Opioids, by State, 2014 and 2017

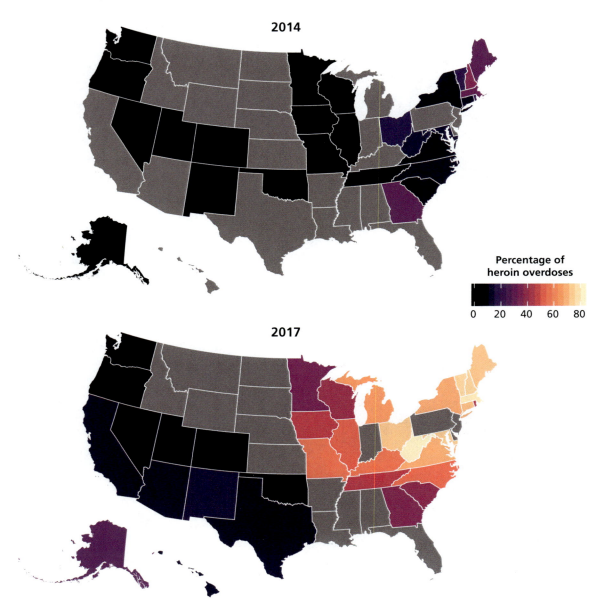

SOURCE: CDC, 2018a.
NOTE: Gray indicates a state that, according to CDC, has only fair overdose reporting and for which the data have therefore been suppressed.

overdoses that contained synthetic opioids, particularly in midwestern states, such as Ohio, and on the East Coast.

Figure 2.7 shows the growth at the state level in the percentage of overdoses due to cocaine that contained synthetic opioids between 2014 and 2017. Here, the color coding on the maps indicates variation at the state level, with purple indicating states with lower percentages of cocaine overdoses that included synthetic opioids, and the green to yellow colors indicating states with higher percentages of overdoses. In 2014, the number of states with cocaine over-

Figure 2.7
Percentage of Cocaine Overdose Deaths That Included Synthetic Opioids, by State, 2014 and 2017

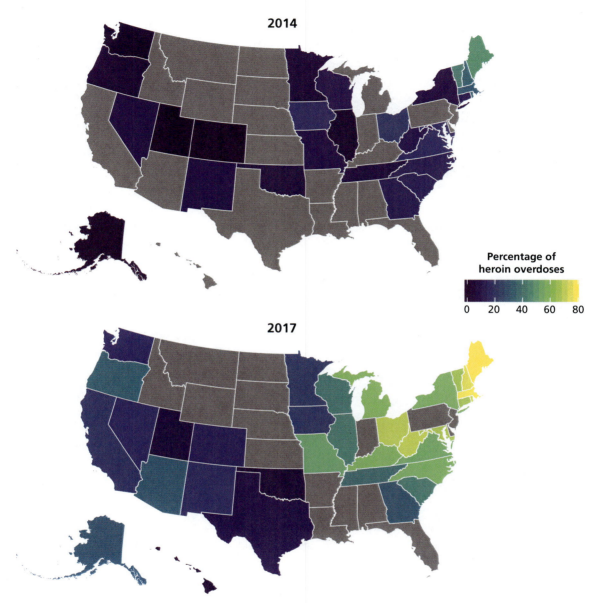

SOURCE: CDC, 2018a.
NOTE: Gray indicates a state that, according to CDC, has only fair overdose reporting and for which the data have therefore been suppressed.

doses that included synthetic opioids was relatively low. By 2017, states with overdoses due to cocaine that contained synthetic opioids were concentrated in the Midwest and on the East Coast. It is unclear why synthetic opioid overdose deaths—even across other drug-poisoning categories, such as heroin and cocaine—are concentrated in the eastern half of the United States. One possible explanation is that fentanyl powder mixes more easily than tablets do with powder heroin, which is more prevalent in the eastern drug markets; whereas, in the West, heroin is often tar or latex (Mars, Bourgois, et al., 2016) and therefore harder to mix with powder forms of synthetic opioids. However, this phenomenon warrants further investigation before we can draw conclusions.

Aggregating deaths up to the state level, we can plot drug overdose trends over time to get a sense of how synthetic opioids have diffused across other drug categories. In Figures 2.8 through 2.10, we show drug overdose death rates at the state level separated by drug class, indicating the share of drug overdose deaths with death certificates that mention synthetic opioids. Again, we have removed annual observations for which overdose deaths were fewer than ten. Therefore, year observations without bars are not true zeros. To avoid double counting, we have excluded drug overdoses with certificates that mention cocaine, heroin, prescription opioids, or psychostimulants; Figures 2.8 through 2.10 show only the rate of synthetic opioid overdoses absent other drugs. The rates of overdoses that involve synthetic opioids displayed in these figures are deflated, given our exclusion of synthetic opioid overdoses that simultaneously mention other drugs. That said, the number of deaths involving *only* synthetic opioids (e.g., those without heroin, cocaine, prescription opioids, or psychostimulants) is growing. Taken together, these trends suggest that some markets are becoming dominated by synthetic opioids.

In Figure 2.8, we show trends in overdoses for New Hampshire—the state with the third-highest rate of overdose deaths due to synthetic opioids in 2017. Here we can see that synthetic opioid–only deaths are even more prevalent than in Ohio (just over 20 per 100,000 population, compared with 12 per 100,000 population). In New Hampshire, heroin and prescription opioid overdoses have continued to decline since 2014, while synthetic opioid overdoses continued to rise year over year. In 2017, in New Hampshire, three-quarters of overdose deaths for

Figure 2.8
Drug Overdose Death Rate per 100,000 Population in 2017: New Hampshire

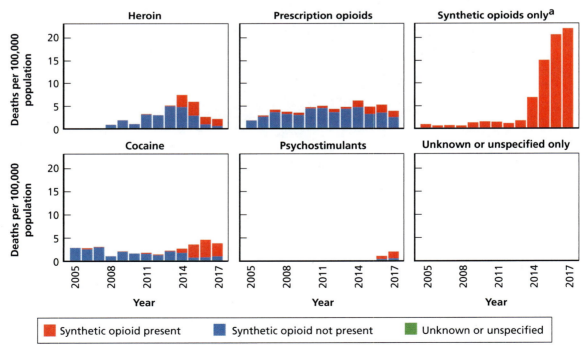

SOURCE: CDC, 2018a.
NOTE: We have excluded years with fewer than ten deaths.
a Excludes cocaine, heroin, prescription opioid, and psychostimulant deaths from synthetic opioids.

heroin, cocaine, or psychostimulants and about one-third of prescription opioids also included synthetic opioids.

In Figure 2.9, we show how overdose deaths in Ohio—the state with the second-highest overdose death rate in 2017 due to synthetic opioids—have changed over time. Synthetic opioid overdose deaths rose year over year starting in 2013. In 2017, fewer heroin overdose deaths were reported for the first time, suggesting that heroin markets in Ohio might be transitioning to synthetic opioids. Of concern is the sharp rise in the share of cocaine, psychostimulant, and prescription opioid overdose deaths with certificates that also mention synthetic opioids. In 2017, three-quarters of heroin, cocaine, or psychostimulant overdoses and about half of prescription opioid overdoses in Ohio included synthetic opioids.

In Figure 2.10, we show overdose deaths in West Virginia—the state with the highest rate of overdose deaths due to synthetic opioids in 2017. This state has long suffered from high rates of prescription opioid abuse and overdose. However, a similar trend toward synthetic opioid overdoses is noted. In 2017, in West Virginia about 80 percent of heroin overdose deaths, 75 percent of cocaine overdose deaths, and 45 percent of prescription opioid overdose deaths involved synthetic opioids.

Figures 2.8 through 2.10 also include fatal overdoses in which a contributing cause of death was unknown or unspecified only. In these cases, coroners and medical examiners could not determine the drug that contributed to the cause of the overdose. As shown in other research, local officials' capacity to accurately assess causes of death varies considerably (Ruhm, 2018).

Figure 2.9
Drug Overdose Death Rate per 100,000 Population in 2017: Ohio

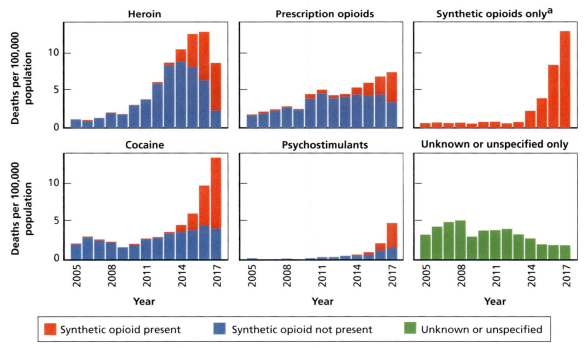

SOURCE: CDC, 2018a.
NOTE: We have excluded years with fewer than ten deaths.
[a] Excludes cocaine, heroin, prescription opioid, and psychostimulant deaths from synthetic opioids.

Figure 2.10
Drug Overdose Death Rate per 100,000 Population in 2017: West Virginia

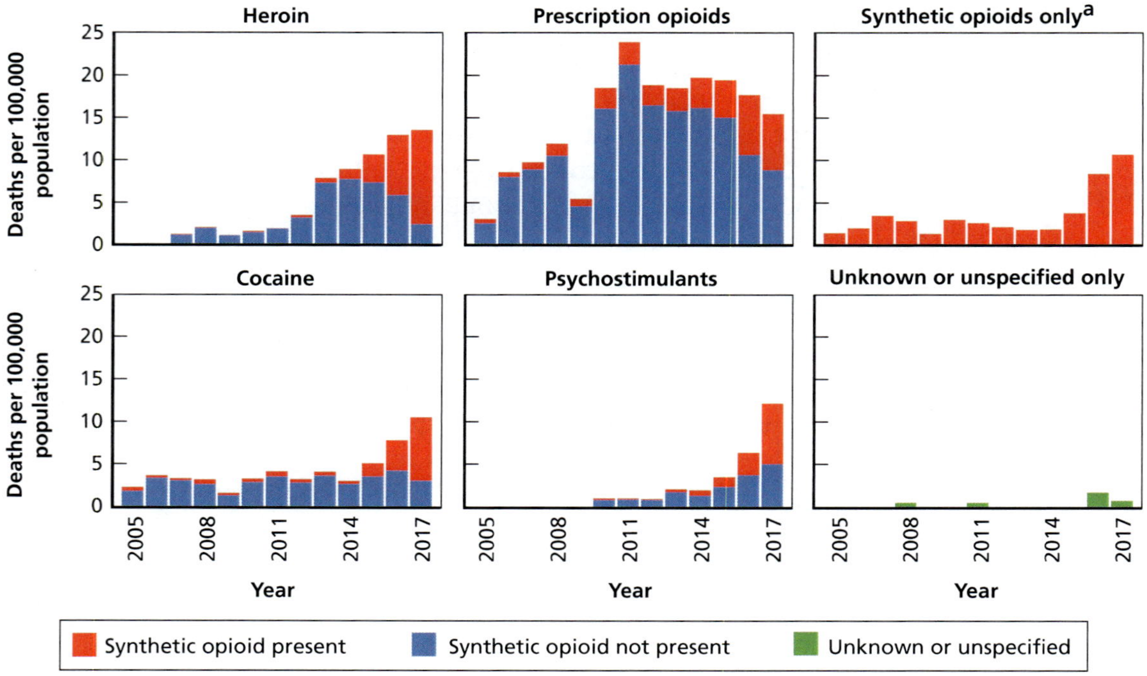

SOURCE: CDC, 2018a.
NOTE: We have excluded years with fewer than ten deaths.
a Excludes cocaine, heroin, prescription opioid, and psychostimulant deaths from synthetic opioids.

More-Granular Targeting Data

The ultimate purpose of understanding the levels and trends in synthetic opioid deaths in states and counties is to enable CBP to improve its targeting of synthetic opioid imports. Although the overdose data presented above show a diffusion of synthetic opioids across other drug classes, we cannot draw strong conclusions from those trends. It appears that drug distributors are mixing fentanyl and other synthetic opioids with heroin, but, from overdose data alone, we are unable to determine where in the supply chain this occurs (e.g., before arrival in the United States or closer to retail markets).

On the other hand, parcels that might contain synthetic opioids shipped by mail or private courier can arrive near retail markets. Therefore, an examination of overdose deaths, by ZIP Code, could help improve targeting efforts at packages arriving at mail facilities.

Limitations

Knowing which ZIP Codes correspond to which counties that report high overdose rates from synthetic opioids does not provide a perfect measure of either demand or supply. State and county hot spots where synthetic opioid deaths are occurring (i.e., reflecting use) might not be perfect proxies for where imported drug shipments are arriving. It is possible, as evidenced by the warehousing phenomenon reported by vendors and indictments (discussed in later chapters), that dealers are located outside areas of high rates of consumption. Thus, the targeting information presented here might not perfectly represent the risk presented by individual parcels at POEs.

Lags in data availability are another limitation to analyses of current trends. CDC does not report overdose deaths in real time. It can take up to a year to have reliable estimates of overdose deaths. ICD-10 codes are another limiting factor of this analysis. CDC data report overdoses only for synthetic opioids, which can include prescribed pharmaceutical fentanyl in addition to other prescribed synthetic opioids, such as tramadol. Knowing precisely the synthetic opioid in question would improve our understanding of its possible source. For the time being, we have relied on the most-recent national data from CDC in order to get a general overview of the synthetic opioid problem. Future efforts that look at overdose death data from state departments of health for 2018 and 2019 might provide further insights into any specific synthetic opioids found in mortality data.

Summary

Analyses of overdose drug data indicate that synthetic opioid deaths are on the rise and reaching exceedingly high levels in some states and especially in some counties. West Virginia, New Hampshire, and Ohio are strongly affected. Understanding the levels and trends of these mortality data, though, reflects only the tip of the iceberg, given the large number of nonfatal drug overdoses in addition to those that result in death. Nonetheless, synthetic opioid deaths appear to be localized to a few areas in a dozen states. These data, especially the associated ZIP Code data, can be used to help CBP (as well as USPIS) target packages from abroad that are destined for markets where synthetic opioids, especially fentanyl, pose the greatest threat.

Unfortunately, overdose death data from CDC are available with a one-year lag. Given how quickly this phenomenon is evolving, 2018 might look different from 2017. To enhance our understanding of this problem, we next turn to supply-side measures. Juxtaposing overdose drug deaths with data derived from drug seizures can provide some additional insights.

CHAPTER THREE

The Evolution of Synthetic Opioid Seizures

The rapid growth in overdose deaths involving synthetic opioids discussed in Chapter Two mirrors supply-side indicators. As noted earlier, the volume of fentanyl seized at IMFs and ECC facilities, as well as at POEs and by border protection, has increased in recent years. Similarly, the number of NSOs—some of which have been detected for the first time—seized by law enforcement has exploded in recent years.

To better understand the national and regional trends in seizures of fentanyl and NSOs, we examined publicly available law enforcement drug seizure data to ascertain several dimensions of this problem of growing concern. First, we assess the publicly available information regarding numbers and POEs of seizures reported by law enforcement agencies. Second, we examine laboratory information on fentanyl and NSO seizures, evaluating state-level trends over time to understand the changes in chemical profiles. This provides a national overview of fentanyl seizures, allowing us to view them alongside overdose death data. Together, these data points allow us to make educated guesses about the supply of these drugs in certain markets, offering law enforcement greater understanding with which to calibrate enforcement strategies and deploy resources.

Understanding the supply-side dimensions of illicit synthetic opioids is increasingly important, given their concealability and potency per gram. As discussed in Chapter One, federal law enforcement believes that fentanyl and other NSOs enter U.S. drug markets by mail from China, as well as from Mexican drug trafficking organizations through traditional smuggling routes across the southwest border. These traditional and unconventional supply routes pose different drug interdiction challenges and policy considerations.

Examining these data points alongside other pieces of information, such as overdose death rates, news reports, and unsealed indictments, allows us to roughly infer the sources of these substances. Knowing whether synthetic opioids arrive via the postal system direct to consumers or dealers near retail markets or are product smuggled over the border is critical for drug interdiction efforts.

In this chapter, we first describe the methods and data sources used in the analysis of spatial and temporal trends of synthetic opioid seizures. We then discuss descriptive findings for each data series. Lastly, we juxtapose our findings with inferred measures of exposure, to offer an overview of the synthetic opioid landscape, providing some insights specific for law enforcement and interdiction.

Methods

Understanding illicit market activities is an inherently challenging task. Classified law enforcement data, such as drug seizure records and laboratory reports, can allow for a richer analysis of the supply of synthetic opioids than publicly available data permit. Here, we have focused our analysis on publicly available information to help construct our understanding of this problem.

We have drawn from publicly available law enforcement reports and congressional testimonies (namely, those from DEA and CBP). Such reports and testimonies provide a general overview of the volume of seizures over time, their likely sources of origin, and illicit actors involved. To understand the evolution in the chemical profiles of synthetic opioids, we utilized laboratory seizure data from NFLIS to provide insights into where and when chemicals enter and exit drug markets. NFLIS systematically collects drug chemistry analysis results and related information from cases analyzed by state, local, and federal forensic laboratories. Partner laboratories examine drugs that law enforcement across the country seize. We paired these data with fatal overdose rates—a crude measure of consumption or exposure—to show how supply of fentanyl and other NSOs relates to the use of synthetic opioids.

Limitations

Before describing the results of this analysis, we briefly underscore several limitations. As mentioned, we are relying on public law enforcement and forensic data, which lack granular details that can further clarify dimensions of this problem. For example, NFLIS seizure case counts are aggregated to the state level and do not report purity nor the proportion of seized fentanyl-containing drugs that are mixed with other drugs, such as heroin.[1]

More importantly, seizure data are not random samples of the supply of drugs. They often contain systematic biases for which we cannot control. They are convenience samples of the supply of fentanyl and other NSOs. Seizures might depend on other factors related to law enforcement priority, capacity, and targeting. Given the rising number of overdose deaths from synthetic drugs, it is likely that law enforcement at every level (federal, state, and local) has prioritized these drug threats in recent years. Therefore, seizure incidence might be confounded by political pressures or policy directives.

Related to that is the fact that drug seizure data do not give us a perfect understanding of illicit drug supply. With traditional drugs, such as cocaine or heroin, it has been challenging to determine the underlying factors that contribute to the increase (or decrease) of seizures from one year to the next (Reuter, 1995). Law enforcement capacity and intensity of efforts to detect and seize illicit drug shipments, as well as smugglers' ability and determination to evade detection, might confound analysis of seizure trends. This is particularly important considering NSOs, which can evade detection because the substance circumvents scheduling controls or because advanced detection methods are not equipped with the latest referent libraries.[2] None-

---

[1]   DEA has produced these figures in the 2018 National Drug Threat Assessment (DEA, 2018c) through 2016. We assess these later.

[2]   Although DEA issued temporary controls over all fentanyl-related substances under its emergency powers (see DEA, 2018b), several other families of non-fentanyl NSOs, such as the Upjohn Company's U-47700 (sometimes referred to in some illicit markets as U-4, pink, and pinky) and Allen and Hanburys' AH-7921, fall outside these regulatory controls.

Toxicology screens of tissue and fluid samples, as well as analytical detection methods used to analyze seizures (e.g., spectroscopy), can test only vis-à-vis a known universe of metabolites or chemicals. These chemical profiles are added to referent libraries once they are detected. It is plausible that early measures of NSOs are biased downward given that ana-

theless, seizure estimates, especially for fentanyl and other NSOs, can indicate the presence of smuggling routes or a drug's presence in markets rather than the volume or intensity of its illicit supply. Data on seizures cannot provide an accurate assessment of the impacts of interdiction efforts. As noted earlier, effects of interdiction efforts can be confounded by other factors.

Findings

Seizure Trends over Time

From analyses of publicly available CBP seizure data (published seizure totals reported in congressional testimony), we note some initial findings. A substantial volume of seizures in FY 2017 that contained fentanyl came from Mexico; however, after we adjusted for reported purity, we found that packages arriving in the postal system from China made up the majority of fentanyl entering the United States seized by law enforcement.

CBP reports seizing synthetic opioids, such as fentanyl, at land POEs and checkpoints on the southwest border. Table 3.1 indicates that, for FY 2017, seizures of fentanyl near or at the border outweighed those at mail and ECC facilities. However, after adjusting for reported purity,[3] we estimate that almost 80 percent of fentanyl seized by CBP in FY 2017 occurred at mail and ECC facilities. Law enforcement and congressional investigations have suggested that these packages originate from China (Permanent Subcommittee on Investigations, 2018;

Table 3.1
Breakdown of Seizures Reported to Contain Fentanyl, Customs and Border Protection, Fiscal Year 2017

Point of Interdiction	Amount Seized, in Kilograms	Number of Seizures	Average Weight of Seizures, in Kilograms	Reported Purity, as a Percentage	Purity-Adjusted Amount, in Kilograms
ECC facilities	110	118	0.93	90	99.0
International mail network	42	227	0.19	90	37.8
Land POEs (southwest border)	388	65	5.97	7.5	29.1
Remainder[a] (presumably border patrol checkpoints)	135			7.5	10.1
Total	675				176

SOURCE: Owen, 2018.

NOTE: Purity at the border is reportedly 5 to 10 percent; here, we use the midpoint.

[a] The remainder is the FY 2017 total (675 kg) minus the amount in reported fentanyl seizures.

---

lytical techniques must be developed and disseminated. For example, one study sponsored by the Office of National Drug Control Policy found that initial screens of urine collected from a sample (n = 175) of emergency department patients in Maryland tested negative for synthetic cannabinoids. The specimens were retested later with an expanded panel, and the researchers found that 25 percent were positive for the presence of more-novel synthetic cannabinoids (Wish et al., 2018).

[3] By adjusting the weight of seizures by purity, we can obtain a more precise measure of the total amount of fentanyl received. Seizures from the border are reportedly very low in purity, suggesting that the gross weight is made up of some

Owen, 2018). That fiscal year, mail facilities documented the largest number of individual seizures, with more than 200 unique parcels. However, the average seizure at IMFs is less than 200 g. Those at ECC facilities are just under 1 kg, the maximum amount generally offered by online vendors outside the United States. Seizures at the southwest border weigh approximately 6 kg, on average.

Seizures at or near the southwest border are reported to be of low purity (DEA, 2018c). News reports and indictments indicate that some of these seized drugs containing fentanyl are pressed into counterfeit pills that resemble prescription medications, such as opioids or benzodiazepines (DEA, 2018c). As a result, we surmise that these seizures are likely destined for retail distribution. Although counterfeit tablets have little fentanyl relative to the rest of the pill's content, they can contain morphine-equivalent amounts comparable to or greater than those in the pharmaceutical products they mimic.

The manufacture, importation, and distribution of counterfeit pills and tablets containing fentanyl and other synthetic opioids present unique challenges to public health and public safety. It combines a traditional drug supply issue with one of trademark infringement. Specifically, drug users consuming these items might be at greater risk of overdose because they might be under the impression that they are using pharmaceutical-grade products of known purity and consistency. Unlike with powders, which are known to vary in quality and purity from bag to bag, those consuming pills might not consider that such tablets contain an unknown quantity of potent synthetic opioids. This is further complicated by the fact that some counterfeit tablets are made to resemble benzodiazepines, not prescription opioids (DEA, 2018c). Further, the counterfeit pill phenomenon might lead to a greater exposure to fentanyl and related substances because pills generally appeal to non–injection drug–using populations, whose opioid tolerance might be lower.

Publicly available reports of CBP seizure data suggest that product entering by mail from China are highly pure powders that are unlikely to be consumed in this form. Given the potency of fentanyl and many of its analogs, these chemicals are often mixed with other drugs, such as heroin; cut with diluents; or pressed with excipients into pills made to resemble prescription medications (Ciccarone, 2017; DEA, 2018c; Mars, Rosenblum, and Ciccarone, 2018).

Nevertheless, smuggling trends might be evolving. In late June 2018, CBP at the Philadelphia POE seized 50 kg of 4-fluoroisobutyryl fentanyl hidden in barrels of iron oxide in a shipment from China (CBP, 2018). CBP noted high purity, which would make this single seizure one of the largest to originate from China.

Types of Chemicals, by Region and over Time

Using publicly available reports from NFLIS, we examined trends in drug seizure data submitted to state and local laboratories for fentanyl and fentanyl-related substances. The data cover the

---

other adulterant or diluent, not fentanyl. This is not to suggest that such seizures are of low *quality*. Fentanyl's potency requires dosing in minute quantities. A counterfeit tablet containing 95-percent filler can exceed the morphine milligram equivalent of a full-strength prescription opioid. For example, if an extended-release oxycodone tablet weighs approximately 120 mg, the estimated amount of fentanyl in a counterfeit tablet from Mexico might be as high as 6 mg, assuming 5-percent purity. This would be a very high dose.

entire United States from 2007 to 2017.[4] During this time period, more than 150,000 counts of fentanyl and fentanyl-related substances have been entered into NFLIS. According to DEA,

> One count represents a single report in the NFLIS-Drug database. Drug cases secured in law enforcement operations (i.e., drug seizures) are submitted to forensic laboratories for analysis. An individual drug case can vary in size, and one case can consist of one or more drug items. Within each item, multiple drugs may be identified and reported. A single report equates to one documented occurrence of a drug. Each report is counted separately and added to the NFLIS-Drug data. (NFLIS, undated, p. 2)

For example, suppose that a retail drug distributor has been detained and law enforcement has seized four bags of powder suspected to be heroin. All four bags are submitted as a single case. Laboratory testing indicates that each bag contains heroin, but two also contain fentanyl. NFLIS data would reflect this as one count of heroin and one count of fentanyl.

Public NFLIS state-year counts are not of individual seizure-level data. Such data would allow us to better understand these seizures, perhaps allowing us to adjust for purity, as well as evaluate drug mixtures (e.g., heroin containing fentanyl) and location. Recent analysis from DEA has reported the combinations of cases (i.e., seizures) that contain fentanyl and other substances for recent years. We calculated the shares of fentanyl cases that contained fentanyl or other drug combinations and display the results in Table 3.2. According to NFLIS data reported by DEA, two-thirds of fentanyl cases contain only fentanyl without the presence of heroin or other drugs. About one-quarter of fentanyl cases contain heroin (DEA, 2018c).

We also analyzed aggregate state-year counts to evaluate trends across states and over time. Table 3.3 shows the numbers of fentanyl-related counts reported by NFLIS in this data series. The vast majority of counts are for fentanyl (79.5 percent), with furanyl fentanyl (5.2 percent), and carfentanil (4.8 percent) showing up as the second- and third-most common chemicals. Another 37 fentanyl-related chemicals were reported in NFLIS but in counts lower than 1,000.

Table 3.2
Fentanyl Cases in NFLIS, as a Percentage

Substance	2014	2015	2016
Fentanyl only	69	70	67
Fentanyl and heroin	25	21	24
Fentanyl and opioids	1	4	4
Fentanyl and other substances	2	2	2
Fentanyl and cocaine	1	1	1
Fentanyl, heroin, and cocaine	1	1	1

SOURCE: DEA, 2018c.
NOTE: Each year's percentages do not sum to 100 because of rounding.

---

[4]   DEA contractors indicate that nearly 100 percent of forensic labs participate, making this more of a census than a sample of the population of laboratory seizure data. However, there is sampling variation in the fact that drug seizures are not randomly collected, making these data a nonrepresentative sample.

Table 3.3
Counts of Fentanyl and Fentanyl-Related Substances Reported to NFLIS for 2007 Through 2017

Chemical	Count
Fentanyl	119,607
Furanyl fentanyl	7,763
Carfentanil	7,155
Acetyl fentanyl	5,562
Acryl fentanyl	2,084
4-fluoroisobutyryl fentanyl	1,646
Cyclopropyl fentanyl	1,445
3-methylfentanyl	1,190
Other[a]	3,929

SOURCE: NFLIS.

[a] The 37 fentanyl-related chemicals reported in NFLIS in counts lower than 1,000.

For 2013 through 2017, NFLIS data show a rapid growth in the number of seizures containing fentanyl and related substances. Likewise, these data allow us to see the chemical evolution of seizures containing fentanyl and other fentanyl-related substances. According to these counts, there is a clear evolution as NSOs are reported with greater frequency. Figure 3.1

Figure 3.1
Drug Seizure Counts for Fentanyl and Fentanyl-Related Substances in the United States in NFLIS for 2007 Through 2017

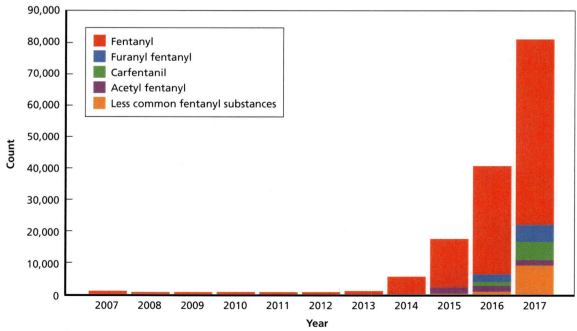

SOURCE: NFLIS public reports.

shows these counts over time. Fentanyl counts remained low and stable through most of the series. However, starting in 2014, there was a noticeable jump, which has continued to accelerate. Counts for fentanyl jumped from 978 in 2013 to more than 59,000 in 2017 (DEA, 2018c). This jump in fentanyl counts mirrors an increase in the counts for other fentanyl-related substances, such as furanyl fentanyl and carfentanil, which were not reported in NFLIS prior to 2015.

Similarly, the number of NSO counts continues to increase year over year. In Figure 3.2, we plot the number of counts for less common fentanyl-related substances over time (i.e., chemicals other than fentanyl, furanyl fentanyl, carfentanil, and acetyl fentanyl). NFLIS reported no counts of NSOs prior to 2014. A handful of instances of butyryl fentanyl were reported in 2014. Counts remained relatively low but exploded from fewer than 900 in 2016 to more than 9,000 in 2017. Between 2014 and 2017, the most–frequently reported fentanyl-related substances were acryl fentanyl (2,084), 4-fluoroisobutyryl fentanyl (1,646), cyclopropyl fentanyl (1,445), and 3-methylfentanyl (1,190).

There is considerable geographic variation of seizures containing fentanyl and fentanyl-related substances. Again, this might be due in part to law enforcement or laboratory practices or capacity. However, parts of New England and Appalachia report the highest number of counts of seizures containing fentanyl or fentanyl-related substances. In Table 3.4, we show the ten states that report the most counts for seizures containing fentanyl or related substances.

Figure 3.2
Drug Seizure Counts for Less Common Fentanyl-Related Substances in the United States in NFLIS for 2007 Through 2017

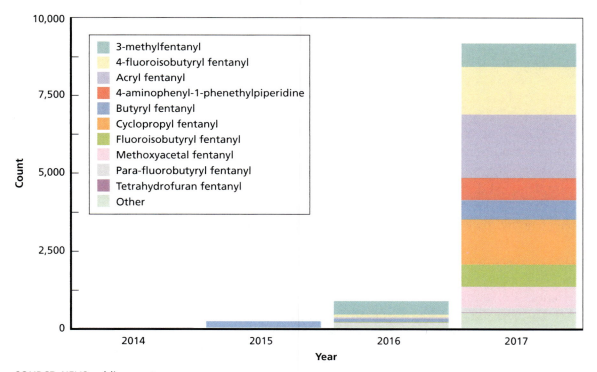

SOURCE: NFLIS public reports.

Table 3.4
**Ten States with the Most Counts
of Fentanyl and Fentanyl-Related
Substances Reported to NFLIS,
2007 Through 2017**

State	Count
Ohio	41,118
Massachusetts	17,631
Pennsylvania	15,899
New Jersey	10,854
Maryland	6,634
New York	6,343
Virginia	6,216
Illinois	5,479
Florida	5,124
New Hampshire	5,083

SOURCE: NFLIS data.

These largely mirror the states with the highest drug overdose death rates involving synthetic opioids (as described in Chapter Two).

However, once we adjusted for population, we noted that Ohio and New Hampshire reported the highest per capita rates of counts containing fentanyl and related substances. In Figure 3.3, we show these trends across the United States over time. Ohio and New Hampshire had high rates as early as 2015. The trend has expanded over time to neighboring states.

When we zoom in on New England and parts of Appalachia, we note an eastward drift in the numbers of counts for fentanyl and fentanyl-related substances (Figure 3.4).

In Table 3.5, we report the 2017 per capita count of NFLIS reports for the above states.

Examining these trends more closely by state and chemical, we see further variation within and across states and over time. In Figures 3.5 and 3.6, we plot these counts for Massachusetts, New Hampshire, New Jersey, and Ohio over time. We note that, in two of these states, fentanyl dominates the counts reported to NFLIS. In New Hampshire and Massachusetts, drug markets contain less variation than in New Jersey and Ohio, where substances other than fentanyl make up more than 40 percent of counts reported to NFLIS in recent years. Massachusetts and New Hampshire also show less variation over time; fentanyl has dominated these markets in recent years. In contrast, fentanyl is less common in New Jersey and Ohio than in the other two states. In New Jersey, furanyl fentanyl is commonly reported. In Ohio, carfentanil is commonly reported.

To help interpret the variation in chemicals across markets, we have calculated the Herfindahl–Hirschman Index (HHI) values for these four states. The HHI is an economic indicator used to calculate how competitive a market is.[5] There are limitations to calculating

---

[5]   The HHI is the sum of squares of the market share of each chemical reported in NFLIS; scores can sum up to 10,000 (meaning that a single chemical makes up 100 percent of the market). For example, if chemical 1 made up 40 percent of

Figure 3.3
Fentanyl and Fentanyl-Related Seizure Counts per 100,000 Persons, 2014 Through 2017

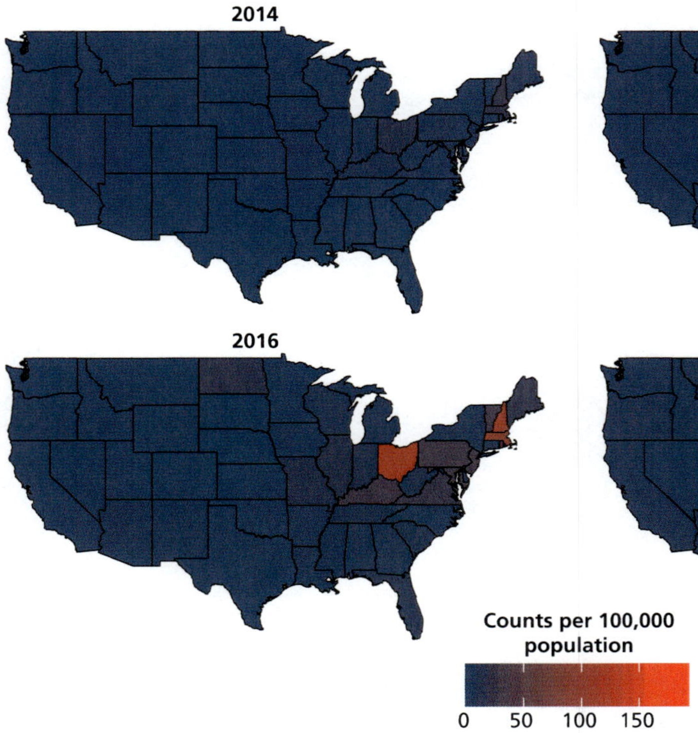

SOURCE: NFLIS public reports.

and interpreting the HHI based on NFLIS counts (as opposed to total pure weight of chemicals), but doing so can quickly show the variation in chemical concentration across different states over time.

In 2013, each state had an HHI of 10,000 because only fentanyl was reported in NFLIS. Over time, Ohio's and New Jersey's HHI scores show that more chemicals are reported in NFLIS in that their HHI scores have declined to about 3,500 and 3,800, respectively. In contrast, New Hampshire and Massachusetts vary less, with HHI scores of about 8,700 and 8,600, respectively. This suggests that those state markets remain less varied in terms of chemicals reported in NFLIS. Figure 3.7 shows the HHIs for these states over time.

This variation among states suggests different supply sources. Given that online vendors from China offer a vast array of NSOs (discussed in greater detail in Chapter Four), buyers in states with greater chemical variation reported in seizure data might be sourcing from the internet. Whereas, states, such as Massachusetts and New Hampshire, that show less chemical variation might be sourcing from single suppliers. Further supporting this hypothesis is that federal law enforcement has detained and indicted fentanyl traffickers in New England with links to Dominican and Mexican drug trafficking organizations (Andersen, 2018; Hernandez, 2016; U.S. Attorney's Office, 2018a, 2018b).

NFLIS seizure counts and three other chemicals each had equal shares of 20 percent of seizure counts, that state's HHI would be $40^2 + 20^2 + 20^2 = 20^2$, or 2,800. The closer a score is to 10,000, the less competition and the greater the domination of a single chemical.

Figure 3.4
Fentanyl and Fentanyl-Related Seizure Counts per 100,000 Persons in Parts of New England and Appalachia, 2014 Through 2017

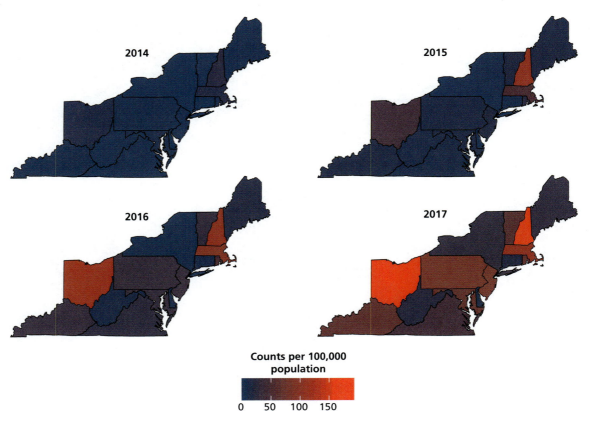

SOURCE: NFLIS public reports.

In this regard, these results suggest that markets dominated by fentanyl alone might be supplied by traditional drug trafficking organizations that utilize common smuggling routes and techniques. In contrast, markets that show greater variation in chemicals might be sourced by the direct-via-mail phenomenon, with individuals purchasing different chemicals from online vendors. CBP strategies might shift detection focus in mail-processing centers to packages destined for areas of high overdoses that report greater chemical variation. Likewise, greater law enforcement efforts (such as intelligence and investigations) should be made to understand how traditional drug trafficking organizations are supplying markets in New England.

Triangulating Laboratory Seizure Data with Fatal Synthetic Opioid Overdose Data

Examining these trends over time and region alongside fatal overdose data enhances our understanding of the dynamics of the supply of fentanyl and related substances. As shown by census division in Figure 3.8, the upward trend in per capita counts of seizures containing fentanyl and other analogs mirrors the change in synthetic opioid overdose death rates reported by CDC. We have indexed overdose deaths to 2013 to show the rate of change through 2017. East North Central, New England, and the Middle Atlantic report increases in the rate of NFLIS counts, as well as an almost-tenfold increase in overdose deaths for synthetic opioids

Table 3.5
2017 Per Capita NFLIS Fentanyl and Fentanyl-Related Counts for Ohio, New England, and Parts of Appalachia

State	Count per 100,000 Persons
Ohio	188.6
New Hampshire	154.8
Massachusetts	104.3
Pennsylvania	77.5
New Jersey	76.1
Maryland	65.6
Rhode Island	64.9
Kentucky	62.5
Vermont	55.7
Virginia	38.6
New York	23.9
Maine	22.5
West Virginia	16.9
Connecticut	13.8
Delaware	8.7

SOURCE: NFLIS data.

over that period. In contrast, the Mountain, Pacific, and West South Central divisions report fewer increases in NFLIS counts, as well as slower rates of increase in synthetic opioid overdose deaths.

Summary

Using publicly available data, we show that seizures containing fentanyl and related substances are increasing over time. In addition, the growing variation of fentanyl analogs reported in NFLIS suggests market evolution. Looking at these data across the United States, we find variation in the supply of synthetic opioids, such as fentanyl. Several regions report high per capita rates of seizures that contain fentanyl and related chemicals. The East North Central and New England census regions, which encompass parts of Appalachia, report the highest per capita rates. The upward trend in NFLIS reports is positively correlated with overdose death rates for synthetic opioids as reported by CDC. Without a doubt, the supply of these substances to domestic drug markets is increasing the harms that drug users experience.

When examining NFLIS data more closely, we note that there is considerable geographic variation in the types of chemicals present. In states in New England, fentanyl predominates in NFLIS observations. In contrast, some states, such as Ohio and some in the Middle Atlan-

Figure 3.5
Fentanyl and Fentanyl-Related Counts in Selected States, 2014 Through 2017

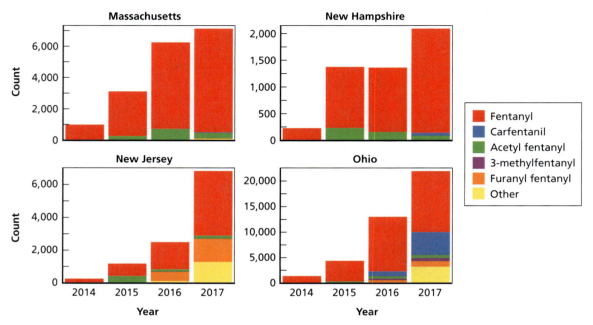

SOURCE: NFLIS public reports.

Figure 3.6
Percentage Distribution of Fentanyl and Fentanyl-Related Counts, Selected States

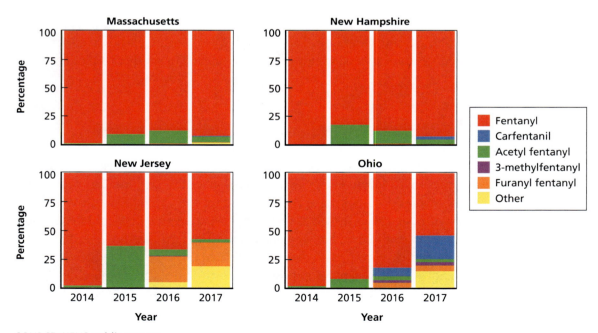

SOURCE: NFLIS public reports.

Figure 3.7
The Herfindahl–Hirschman Index Comparing Concentrations of Fentanyl Seizure Counts in Selected States, 2013 Through 2017

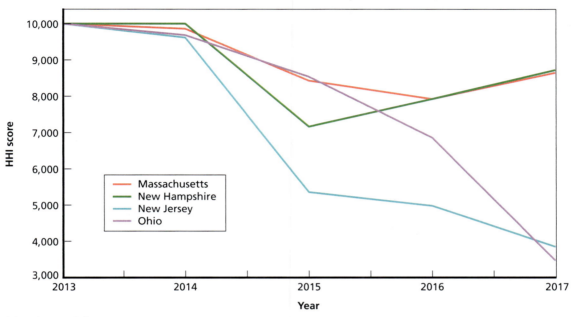

SOURCE: NFLIS data.

tic, show greater variation in the types of chemicals reported. For example, about 45 percent of counts in Ohio in 2017 were fentanyl analogs. Assuming that testing protocols and referent libraries do not vary much among laboratories that report to NFLIS, the distinction in the types of chemicals reported by laboratories in different states suggests that these markets might be supplied by different sources. In the case of markets in New England, the lack of variation in chemicals suggests fewer suppliers or entrants to the market. In these cases, markets might be supplied by more-traditional drug trafficking organizations. States that report greater variation in seizure data might be supplied by online vendors from China that offer a multitude of ever-changing analogs.

That said, limitations to this analysis remain. Without having individual-level seizure observations, we cannot determine the total amounts of fentanyl and fentanyl-related substances that are seized in the United States. Unable to assess the drug mixtures of seizures, we reproduce data reported by DEA, which show that about 70 percent of seizures containing fentanyl are absent any other drug. Only about one-quarter of fentanyl-related seizures contain heroin. Without knowing whether seizures are at the wholesale level or retail level, we cannot assess where in the supply chain the mixing is occurring.

Assessing illicit market activity based on unprivileged public data provides only a rough insight into the evolution of the supply of illicit synthetic opioids. Our analysis here suggests variation in supply sources, with chemicals from China concentrated in some states but perhaps not in others. Drug law enforcement efforts should be tailored to these different sources of supply. Understanding the variation on the ground can improve law enforcement's response.

Figure 3.8
Per Capita NFLIS Counts for Fentanyl and Synthetic Opioid Overdose Death Rates, by Census Division

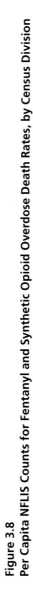
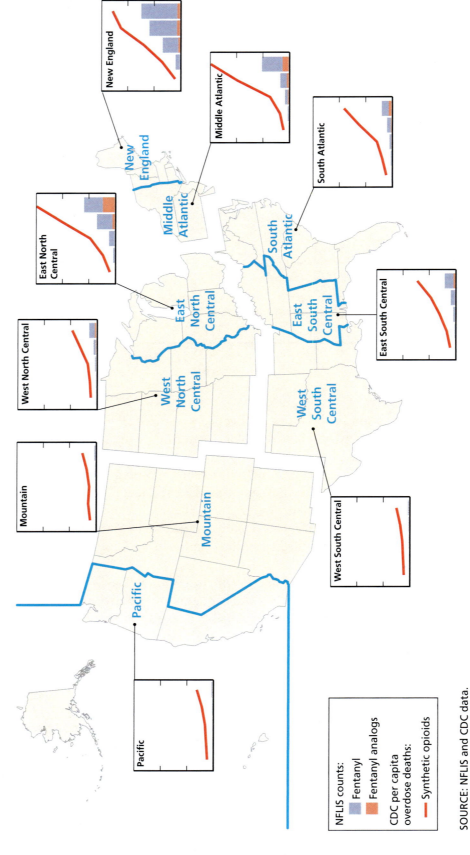

SOURCE: NFLIS and CDC data.

NOTE: The upward trend in NFLIS counts of seizures containing fentanyl and other analogs per 100,000 population (bars) mirrors the change in synthetic opioid overdose death rates reported by CDC, indexed to 2013 (2013 = 100) (lines). The tick marks are at 0, 500, 1,000, and 1,500. The horizontal axes are years: 2013, 2014, 2015, 2016, 2017.

CHAPTER FOUR

Supply and Trafficking Methods for Synthetic Opioids

As discussed in other chapters, fentanyl and NSOs are illicitly imported via the legitimate international mail system and private ECCs, as well as smuggled across both the northern and southern U.S. borders. Law enforcement reports suggest that some amount of fentanyl trafficked over the border with Mexico might be mixed with heroin (DEA, 2018c). Analysis of seizures reported by CBP for FY 2017, after being adjusted for purity, suggest that the majority of fentanyl that is seized arrives from China through IMFs and ECCs. Fentanyl and other NSOs present a new challenge to drug law enforcement. The potency (as measured in morphine-equivalent doses) of many of these chemicals can be orders of magnitude greater than that of morphine (Vardanyan and Hruby, 2014). Furthermore, their availability through online vendors makes these substances attractive alternatives for drug distributors and some end users. The potency-to-weight ratio gives fentanyl and NSOs a strategic and economic advantage to drug trafficking organizations, which often go to extensive lengths to conceal illicit shipments.

Understanding the share of fentanyl and other NSOs entering the United States, as well as the methods used by suppliers and drug trafficking organizations to circumvent CBP detection, is crucial to interdiction efforts. Estimating seizure rates for traditional drugs has been a challenge for drug law enforcement for the past 50 years.[1] Absent reliable estimates of the total amount produced, we are unable to estimate the share of fentanyl and other NSOs that arrive in the United States that comes from China or Mexico. As reported in Chapter Three, most of the purity-adjusted fentanyl that is interdicted by CBP arrives from China via the post and express consignment systems.

Given the challenges of estimating these shares, especially when facing data limitations, we were tasked with cataloging and describing the various delivery and supply methods employed by suppliers of fentanyl and other NSOs. Analyzing production from Mexico, which is often linked to drug trafficking organizations, is not feasible at this time given the lack of data.[2] However, information on online vendors offers substantial insights into those actors and their distribution strategies. In this chapter, we describe the online retailing of fentanyl and related substances from vendors overseas. These online retail data provide some insights into supply and trafficking mechanisms by suppliers from Asia. We have supplemented this with

---

[1] Seizure rates can be measured as a share of the numerator (drug shipments interdicted) over the denominator (the total supply in a given period). Law enforcement collects data on the numerator (drug shipments) in seizure records, but measuring total amount supplied (the denominator—i.e., the amount that is presumed to arrive in U.S. drug markets plus the amount interdicted) is an imprecise measure. With plant-based drugs, scholars and law enforcement would approximate that amount using heroin production potential as measured by satellite imagery of poppy fields in drug-producing countries. Synthesis of opioids makes estimating production potential extremely difficult.

[2] Mexican seizure data were unavailable to analyze fentanyl trafficking in that country.

additional qualitative information from unsealed federal indictments and public government reports.

Analysis of individual drug seizures would enhance the findings here. This analysis suggests that online vendors recognize the illegality of the supply of many of these chemicals, as well as the risk that law enforcement or postal inspectors will intercept their packages. They describe their product in detail to potential clients, including purity and effects. Online vendors discuss several shipping and supply strategies used to circumvent customs authorities while offering free reshipments on packages that are seized. Presumably, these details are used to offer assurances to potential customers that orders will arrive undetected.

This chapter discusses the methods and findings of our analysis of fentanyl and NSOs sold online through vendor webpages and marketplaces accessible on the surface web.[3] We discuss their product pages and efforts to conceal shipments.

Methods

This task presents unique challenges. For obvious reasons, drug trafficking organizations do not openly discuss their concealment methods, requiring analysts to examine seizure data and other law enforcement intelligence to get a better understanding of such practices. We used publicly available data, as well as our unique data set of online marketplaces offering synthetic opioids. Unlike traditional drug trafficking organizations, which go to great lengths to hide their supply methods, online vendors openly discuss some of their supply and concealment practices, at least in general terms. This could be in part to the fact that fentanyl and other NSOs that originate overseas are offered openly online and supplied via legitimate transport and commercial systems. Vendors might offer such information to assure customers that their orders will bypass authorities.

Approaching this task, we conducted web scrapes of three surface-web online marketplaces,[4] conducted an in-depth analysis of eight of the most popular surface-web vendor websites (as measured by search engine page rank), and reviewed public government reports and unsealed DOJ indictments from ongoing criminal conspiracies in China.

Marketplace Data
To supplement the data collection and analysis, we scraped available data (e.g., company name and information, details on products) from individual product listings found on three online

---

[3] We focus on the surface web instead of the dark web, which requires more technical knowhow to access, because many online vendors from overseas operate using websites that are readily accessible via common search engines. Dark-web vendors are increasingly reluctant to offer product that purportedly contains fentanyl or other analogs (Townsend, 2018). Ongoing analysis of listings on some dark-web marketplaces has shown a steep decline for those mentioning synthetic opioids starting in April 2018 (Lamy and Daniulaityte, 2018), although researchers note that retailers might have adapted to the ban by using alternative code words to indicate product containing fentanyl or other NSOs. The retail of fentanyl through the dark web might differ substantially in other important ways from that of other traditional drugs of abuse or novel psychoactives. DEA has discussed U.S.-based fentanyl distributors that import powdered fentanyl from China to press into counterfeit pills for retail on the dark web (DEA, 2018c).

[4] These are akin to eBay or Alibaba. Individual sellers can use these platforms to offer their products.

marketplaces.[5] Unsealed indictments and media reports indicate that buyers in the United States will find online vendors of fentanyl and other synthetic opioids on the surface web (as opposed to the dark web, which requires more-sophisticated and -technical knowhow to access).

We used the following four steps to scrape and build a supplemental data series that allowed us to analyze a cross-section of products containing fentanyl.

Step 1: Identify Online Vendors

In October 2018, we used a search engine to identify marketplaces for fentanyl. We searched the web only in English. Some of the search results were not vendors or marketplaces but news stories about buying fentanyl online. We focused on the most-popular marketplaces by limiting our scraping analysis to websites found in the first two pages of returns (ten results, not counting ads).

An initial assessment of vendor websites indicated that scraping several sites would be infeasible given the unique coding required to scrape each site and because of the risk that a site would be taken offline without notice. Instead, our scraping focused on three online vendors, which we call marketplace 1, marketplace 2, and marketplace 3. These marketplace websites provided more-uniform item entries than those on individual websites do, allowing us to obtain information on company name, location, product offered, product descriptions, and shipping.

Step 2: Identify Search Terms and Scrape the Product Listings

We first identified search terms to return fentanyl-related products from marketplace vendors. We scraped using a combination of packages in the programming language Python to extract relevant product listings from each of the three marketplaces. Once scraped, the data were organized into a data-frame structure for further analysis.

Step 3: Clean the Data

After having been scraped, data sometimes required additional cleaning. This is particularly true for text-based fields that contain long string or character values. Data cleaning was done primarily in Microsoft Excel.

Step 4: Analyze the Data

Cleaned and organized data were then submitted for further analysis. Findings are presented in "Findings" later in this chapter.

Vendor Websites

In addition to analyzing product listings from marketplaces in Asia, we wanted to examine specific online fentanyl vendor webpages. Assuming the perspective of a potential customer, we used online search engines to find vendors that claimed to distribute fentanyl and other NSOs. The team focused on the most-popular vendors by limiting the analysis to websites

---

[5] Web scraping is a common practice that uses automation to extract data from a website, allowing text-based data to be cleaned and analyzed.

found in the first two pages of returns. When we searched in November 2018, this returned eight unique vendors.[6]

As mentioned above, scraping these individual sites proved to be problematic. Instead, we undertook a more qualitative approach to data extraction and analysis by reading vendor "about us" sections, as well as relevant shipping and payment policy pages, frequently asked question (FAQ) sections, and other relevant pages, to gather information on location, shipping techniques, products offered, and payment methods accepted. We prioritized information on shipping methods and strategies discussed on vendor sites.

Unsealed Indictments and Public Government Reports

Our analysis was supplemented by information gleaned from unsealed criminal indictments released by DOJ related to Chinese nationals operating online outlets that promote and distribute fentanyl and related substances. In addition, we parsed information from publicly available government reports detailing the supply strategies and techniques of online vendors. We cite these sources in the "Findings" section later in this chapter.

Limitations

Although the work presented in this chapter is novel, we note that many unknowns still surround the synthetic opioid threat. Further research could help confirm or supplement the findings discussed here. There are limitations to this approach. For example, we conducted searches only in English. Data on product listings from marketplaces might not truly reflect what products are being offered online or what buyers in the United States are ordering. We did not randomly sample from websites but instead assumed the perspective of a potential buyer interested in synthetic opioids. Our specific product search terms might not have captured all fentanyl listings that potential customers saw or sought. Vendor sites would sometimes go down or be removed from search returns. There is also concern that specific vendor sites might be scams, intentionally designed to extract funds from potential customers without actually shipping any product. There is no way for us to verify the veracity of online vendors or any claims made by websites. The findings from online vendors should therefore be interpreted with caution, especially given that sites could be fraudulent or taken offline. Analysis here might become outdated or limited to this one point in time (November and December 2018).

Findings

Online Marketplaces

We identified three online marketplaces where vendors listed fentanyl and related products. Online marketplaces are not unique vendor websites but online distribution platforms that allow sellers to list products. This is sometimes known as business-to-business or business-to-consumer commerce. We identified two marketplaces hosted in China and one hosted in India. We included the one marketplace from India to give further insights into the distribution of fentanyl and related products from overseas. To our knowledge, this is the first unclas-

---

[6]   Unique online vendor webpages can sometimes go down or be closed by authorities. At the time of this writing, we had found and analyzed eight.

sified quantitative analysis of such marketplaces and the first to explore the role of product that might originate from India.

Vendors are sometimes prohibited from selling products that marketplace operators have banned. We identified about 280 unique product listings when we ran our scraping analysis in October 2018. Table 4.1 provides a breakdown of the number of listings found on each marketplace, as well as the number of listings that mention some details on product formulation (e.g., powder, pills, or patches). The Indian marketplace listed the most products. Powder and patch formulations were reported more frequently in the titles of product listings, suggesting that some of the products offered might be diverted pharmaceutical products. Pill formulations were mentioned infrequently. It is impossible to tell at this time whether these were legitimate pharmaceutical-grade products that were diverted to online markets by third parties or whether pharmaceutical manufacturers themselves were selling these products out the backdoor. In either case, such activity violates international drug accords.

Individual listings contain a substantial amount of information. In Figure 4.1, we reproduce a screenshot from each of the marketplaces. Note the amount of information provided to potential customers. This includes information on the substances themselves, such as their purity and quality, as well as shipping methods, including delivery times and packaging aimed at avoiding detection.

From the scraped data, we were able to evaluate individual product listings, extracting company names and searching for words or terms indicating supply mechanisms or concealment strategies. Table 4.2 shows a frequency of selected targeted search terms for product listings.

Most product listings did not include targeted search terms because the pages lacked detailed product descriptions. In terms of products sold on each, marketplace 2 had the most listings for synthetic opioids other than fentanyl (as measured by our search terms for carfentanil and several other NSOs). However, for shipment methods, listings referred to EMS (i.e., the postal service) twice as often as ECCs, such as FedEx or DHL. This supports what unsealed federal indictments mentioned about online vendors' stated preference for using the international postal system over private couriers (*United States of America v. Fujing Zheng*, 2018). The recent USPS Inspector General's report also points to several factors that make the international postal system attractive to online vendors, including the overwhelming number of items processed by USPS and Fourth Amendment protections against warrantless search and seizure (Office of Inspector General, 2018).

Table 4.1
Breakdown of Online Marketplace Product Listings

Marketplace	Unique Product Listings	Research Chemical	Powder	Patch	Injection	Pill or Tablet
1	149	9	47	54	2	1
2	74	10	14	1	0	3
3	58	6	1	9	0	5
Total	281	25	62	64	2	9

Figure 4.1
Examples of Product Listings for Fentanyl and Related Substances on Three Online Marketplaces

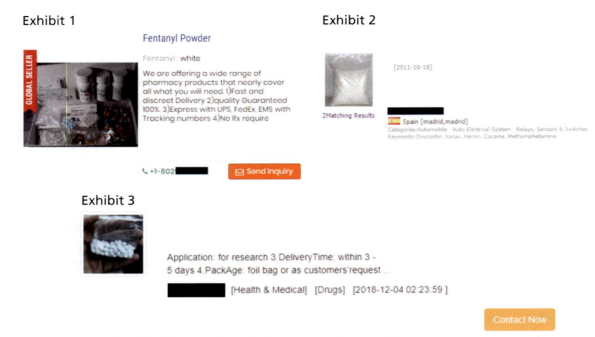

NOTE: We have redacted individual vendor and seller names and contact information.

For packaging and concealment methods discussed on product listings, vendors mention bags and aluminum with the greatest frequency. Several discuss discreet packaging methods, perhaps to assure potential buyers. In several cases, these refer to plastic or aluminum foil bags. These are discussed in terms of how product is shipped, in containers designed to ensure discreet delivery. In several instances, product listings describe the possibility of shipping in 25-kg drums for bulk orders.

In terms of payment methods, Bitcoin and Western Union were discussed with similar frequency.

The information extracted from scraping product listings also included names of companies. In Table 4.3, we report the ten companies with the most product listings, in descending order of the number of product listings they have. The top listed company, vendor 1, had 11 unique product listings for items containing fentanyl or related substances. According to its company page listing, it specializes in "exporting high quality Research chemical [sic]" using its own in-house chemists."

From the scrape analysis, we found 234 unique companies or listings by unique individuals. Most companies or unique individual listings were for just one item or product that contained fentanyl or related substances. Many of these firms maintain their own websites, although several share templates and organizational structures, suggesting that a single manufacturer might be using multiple shell companies to offer and distribute product. Unsealed federal indictments speak to multiple company names and website mirrors linked to the same manufacturers (see, e.g., *Zheng*, 2018). Those monitoring fentanyl production in China have noted the same elsewhere (O'Connor, 2017).

Table 4.2
Substances, Shipping, Packaging, and Payment Mentions in Product Listings

Item	Search Term	Marketplace			Total
		1	2	3	
Substance					
Carfentanil		2	7	0	9
Furanyl fentanyl		1	8	0	9
U-47700		1	3	0	4
U-49900		1	3	0	4
Shipping					
DHL	dhl	3	2	0	5
FedEx	fedex	2	2	1	5
Express Mail Service	ems	6	3	1	10
UPS	ups	2	2	0	4
Mail	mail	3	27	7	37
Packaging and concealment					
Bag (e.g., plastic, foil)	bag	1	13	0	14
Drum (container)	drum	0	3	0	3
Bulk shipment	bulk	8	1	3	12
Discreet	discreet, discrete	7	1	7	15
Wholesale	wholesale	4	0	1	5
Aluminum	alumi	1	14	0	15
Payment					
Bitcoin	bitcoin	2	2	0	4
Western Union	western	2	2	0	4
Payment	pay	4	2	0	6

Vendor Websites

To expand on these marketplace findings, we decided to conduct more in-depth assessments of unique online retailers that specialize in or offer fentanyl and other related products. We searched only in English and limited our analysis to vendors that showed up in the first two pages of returns, assuming that a typical buyer would not go beyond the second page of results. Search results suggest that an individual seeking to buy fentanyl online can find a handful of vendors immediately in the first page of returns.

We identified eight vendors selling fentanyl or related products. From these websites, we gathered information regarding available products and other relevant information from the companies' "about us" sections, shipment and payment policies, FAQs, and other relevant parts of vendor sites. This examination of vendor sites yielded some important findings. Most offer various research chemicals, such as synthetic cannabinoids, novel benzodiazepines, analge-

Table 4.3
The Ten Marketplace Sellers with the Most Product Listings

Vendor	Number of Product Listings
1	11
2	5
3	5
4	4
5	4
6	3
7	3
8	3
9	2
10	2

sics, and other new psychoactive substances. Only two sold exclusively fentanyl or related substances in various formulations (i.e., patches, pills, lozenges, powders). All but one had live chat boxes in which customers could communicate with sales representatives. Most promoted discretion and privacy, as well as methods to avoid customs detection. All but one mentioned warehouses in the United States, Europe, or Australia.

Table 4.4 is a comparative overview of the eight sites, including information on categories of substances and shipment methods. Most vendor websites recognize that they operate on the legal margins, but they assume no legal risk. Several indicate in their FAQs or other policy pages that they do not sell or export prohibited products but that it is the buyer's responsibility to determine whether the product is permitted in the receiving country prior to ordering. This finding was confusing because several vendors reported to be outside of China. Most vendors indicated the use of warehouses overseas for the purposes of avoiding customs at ports of entry. In several cases, vendors would note that shipments to Europe would originate from facilities on that continent. This was also true for several webpages that mentioned warehouses in the United States.[7]

Using the Internet Corporation for Assigned Names and Numbers (ICANN) domain-lookup service WHOIS (WHOIS, undated), we were able to include information on when each vendor registered its domain uniform resource locator (URL), as well as the web host with which it registered. Vendors conceal their identities by using third-party client registration companies. With the exception of one vendor's, these URLs were registered within the past few years.

Vendors are very customer oriented. Most are easy to navigate and professional looking. In addition to live chat interfaces, vendors might include contact information via WhatsApp, text, or email. Websites offered assurances to potential customers that their products were of

---

[7] Warehousing inventory closer to demand reduces the risks and costs associated with product crossing international boundaries. This poses considerable challenges to drug law enforcement, especially CBP, which screens packages entering the country. Once in the domestic mail system, USPIS assumes jurisdiction.

high quality and that their distribution systems were legitimate, as opposed to other potential online scams. One vendor linked to a promotional video explaining the benefits of ordering through its website. All reported quality customer service. Some even posted customer reviews of products, although several were repetitive or nonsensical, suggesting to us that they might have been falsified.

Some vendors guarantee delivery, with many offering free reshipment should the package get lost, stolen, or seized by customs. To entice potential customers, some vendors mention or include free samples on eligible orders. Only two boasted that they had high rates of success circumventing customs, although one noted that packages sent to Scandinavia encountered some trouble. In terms of shipping, vendors send product through the international postal system (EMS), as well as by private consignment carriers (e.g., FedEx, DHL). Some indicated a preference for EMS or USPS, and, in one case, the vendor would deny free reshipments if seized by a private courier of the customer's choosing. With regard to packaging mechanisms, most mentioned discreet or plain packaging, such as unmarked envelopes, to circumvent customs. Only one elaborated on what that entailed, citing double-lined plastic bags or aluminum foil.

Only one vendor indicated that the customer could choose partial delivery (e.g., split orders into multiple packages) at checkout, and five indicated that bulk or wholesale orders were available upon request. Several vendors suggested that clients contact customer service for unique orders or further questions. There was no explicit indication of what was considered bulk, but, depending on the chemical in question, product could be purchased in amounts ranging from as low as 1 g to as much as 1 kg across websites. One vendor indicated that customers should contact the vendor regarding packages heavier than 3 kg. Bulk discount prices were offered, with orders on larger quantities costing less per gram.

Vendors preferred wire transfers or cryptocurrency (Bitcoin being the most frequently recommended). One accepted gift cards from U.S. customers (including Amazon or Steam credit, asking the client to submit photos of the card's serial and activation numbers after placing the order). None claimed to accept credit cards.

Product listings on vendor sites varied considerably in terms of detail and description. In Figures 4.2 through 4.5, we show screenshots of product listings for a handful of synthetic opioids that vendors offered. In some cases, vendors would provide technical information regarding purity, chemical name, price, quantity, and shipping and payment details. Several included photos of the substance.

Triangulating with Federal Indictments

To verify some of the findings from our supplemental analysis of marketplace listings and vendor websites, we gathered information from unsealed federal indictments of ongoing criminal conspiracies linked to manufacturers and distributors in China. These indictments provide extensive and detailed pieces of evidence, as described by federal prosecutors and law enforcement, on the operations of fentanyl manufacturers and distributors. We drew in particular from two cases: *United States v. Zhang*, filed January 2018 in the District of North Dakota, and *Zheng*, filed August 2018 in the Northern District of Ohio.

According to information from prosecutors, the Zheng criminal organization maintained a rotating set of online storefronts that used multiple URLs, advertising 100-percent guarantee of product delivery and reshipment if seized by customs. Websites touted warehouses in North America and Europe able to circumvent screening at the POE. The indictment goes on to note

Table 4.4
Descriptive Information About Vendor Websites

Feature	Vendor 1	Vendor 2	Vendor 3	Vendor 4	Vendor 5	Vendor 6	Vendor 7	Vendor 8
URL creation date	October 2016	January 2016	January 2018	August 2016	November 2017	February 2018	July 2017	April 2014
Web host or registrar	Shinjiru Technology	NameSilo	OnlineNIC	Shinjiru MSC Sdn Bhd	Namecheap	Namecheap	Tucows	Public Domain Registry
Search result page	1	1	1	1	1	2	2	2
About us page	Yes	Yes	Yes	Yes	Yes	Yes	Yes	No
Shipping or payment page	No	Yes	Yes	Yes	No	No	No	Yes
FAQ page	Yes	Yes	No	No	No	No	No	Yes
Product categories	Benzodiazepines, research chemicals, analgesics, cannabinoids	Research chemicals, cannabinoids, dissociatives, ecstasy, analgesics, prescription drugs	Fentanyl (powders, citrate, pills, patches), carfentanil, oxycodone	Research chemicals, cannabinoids, anxiolytics, fentanyl powder, pill presses	Fentanyl (sublingual, patches, powder, citrate)	Cannabinoids, research chemicals, psychedelics, fentanyl	Cannabinoids, cocaine, stimulants, fentanyl, opioids	Stimulants, cannabinoids, research chemicals, fentanyl
Live chat	Yes	Yes	Yes	Yes	Yes	Yes	Yes	No
Purported location	Ukraine	United States and Europe	Ukraine and United States	Undetermined	United States (Virginia)	United States (Massachusetts)	China	China
Overseas warehousing	Not stated	Australia	United States and Europe	Australia, Spain, United States, and Russia	Not stated	Netherlands	Yes	United States
Shipping methods	USPS or EMS preferred but also DHL and FedEx	UPS, FedEx, TNT Express, and DHL preferred; does not offer EMS	USPS or EMS preferred but also DHL and FedEx	UPS, DHL, FedEx, TNT Express, and EMS	Not stated	Not stated	USPS, EMS, and DHL	DHL, EMS, FedEx, TNT Express, Aramex, Blueair, Express Rox

Table 4.4—Continued

Feature	Vendor 1	Vendor 2	Vendor 3	Vendor 4	Vendor 5	Vendor 6	Vendor 7	Vendor 8
Shipping time	8–10 days standard	3 days to United States, United Kingdom, Australia, or Canada	4–7 days express	3–7 days express	Fast	Not stated	Fast	4–7 days
Partial delivery	Not stated	Not stated	Not stated	Offers partial delivery	Not stated	Not stated	Not stated	Not stated
Free reshipping	Yes, limit 1	Yes	Yes, limit 1	Yes, plus double order	Not stated	Not stated	Yes	For insured orders
Bulk shipping	Wholesale orders available	Not stated	Wholesale orders available	Not stated	Wholesale orders available	Wholesale orders available	Wholesale orders available	Available with inquiry
Delivery tracking	Available	Not available for privacy reasons	Available	Available	Available	Not stated	Available	Not stated
Packaging mechanisms	Discreet, plain packaging	"Stealth" packaging	Discreet, plain packaging	Strong courier box with double-lined plastic bag or "robust" aluminum foil	Discreet shipping	Not stated	Discreet containers	Not stated
Claimed delivery success rate	Not stated	Not stated, but higher interdiction risk noted in Scandinavia	Not stated	100% in Europe	Not stated	Not stated	Not stated	Not stated
Payment method	Wire transfer, bank transfer, or Bitcoin	Gift card, wire transfer, or Bitcoin	Wire transfer or Bitcoin	CryptoCoin, MoneyGram, bank wire	Bitcoin	Bitcoin	Bank transfer, Bitcoin, or MoneyGram	Bank transfer, wire transfer, or Bitcoin

Figure 4.2
Product Listing for Penta-Fentanyl

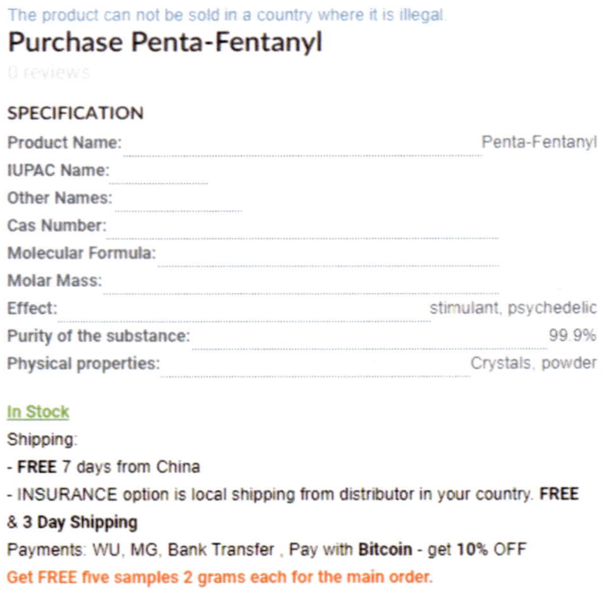

The product can not be sold in a country where it is illegal.

Purchase Penta-Fentanyl

0 reviews

SPECIFICATION

Product Name:	Penta-Fentanyl
IUPAC Name:	
Other Names:	
Cas Number:	
Molecular Formula:	
Molar Mass:	
Effect:	stimulant, psychedelic
Purity of the substance:	99.9%
Physical properties:	Crystals, powder

In Stock
Shipping:
- **FREE** 7 days from China
- INSURANCE option is local shipping from distributor in your country. **FREE**
& 3 Day Shipping
Payments: WU, MG, Bank Transfer , Pay with **Bitcoin** - get **10%** OFF
Get FREE five samples 2 grams each for the main order.

SOURCE: Vendor 8.

that sales representatives from the Zheng criminal organization used various forms of secure private messaging, including WhatsApp.

To avoid detection, investigators noted, the Zheng organization would falsify customs declarations (mislabeling exports as "sebacic acid," "hydrogen peroxide resin," "Portland cement," "fire retardant," or "azelaic acid"), use freight forwarders, ship from warehouses in the destination country, and conceal narcotics within bulk cargo that contained legal goods. The indictment went into extensive detail about the Zheng warehouse facility in Woburn, Massachusetts, which was a chemical company used to import product from China in hidden bulk shipments. This facility in the United States was then used to forward shipments to buyers across the country.

The indictment noted the organization's expertise in avoiding seizure, knowing which customs facilities to target. A sales representative of the organization responding in an email to a prospective customer stated, "[I]f you have an address in Eastern US state, that would be best, cos [sic] New York customs is easiest to pass." According to email exchanges with prospective buyers, the organization noted its use of heat-sealed aluminum foil bags with markings to make it appear as if the chemical had been shipped in nitrogen-sealed containers.[8] All of this was to avoid detection and interference by customs agents at ports of exit and entry. To spread detection and interdiction risk, the Zheng organization would also sometimes divide shipments into multiple packages. The organization would often ship using EMS but also used DHL and FedEx.

---

[8] According to the indictment, "certain chemicals are transported in nitrogen sealed containers. For these chemicals, opening a nitrogen sealed bag would render them inert and thus valueless. [The defendant suggested,] 'Yes. This way [customs] won't check it.'"

Figure 4.3
Product Listing for Furanyl Fentanyl

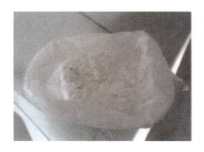

buy Furanyl fentanyl Online

$200.00 - $1,900.00

IUPAC: N-(1-(2-phenylethyl)-4-piperidinyl)-N-

CAS:

Molecular Weight:

Molecular Formula:

Quantity in Grams
Choose an option ▾

SOURCE: Vendor 2.
NOTE: The quantity offered in the dropdown menu ranged from 10 to 200 g.

Interestingly, vendors responded to Chinese drug controls. When the Chinese government controlled acetyl fentanyl in October 2015, the Zheng organization explained that it replaced its inventory with a legal alternative, furanyl fentanyl.

In Chapter Three, we examined NFLIS fentanyl counts and suggested that variation in chemicals reported in laboratories might indicate variation in supply channels. The analysis above shows that fentanyl alone makes up almost all the counts reported in NFLIS, whereas, in Ohio and New Jersey, fentanyl makes up about half the counts. The former suggests a single source, whereas the latter suggests multiple sources of fentanyl. Here, to further test this hypothesis, we examined federal legal action in New England and Ohio.

Initially, the team attempted to scan the unsealed indictments in the Public Access to Court Electronic Records (PACER) system for distributing or trafficking fentanyl. However, the limitations presented in searching prevented us from extracting offenses specific to fentanyl (instead of all schedule II drugs). With more time and resources, a proper scan of PACER might be possible. Instead, we accessed LexisNexis to search the Federal News Service (Federal News Service, undated), a news information service that reports on press releases across the federal government. We searched the service for DOJ press releases related to fentanyl trafficking or distribution in 2017 and 2018. We used the following Boolean search query: (traffick*

Figure 4.4
Product Listing for Carfentanil

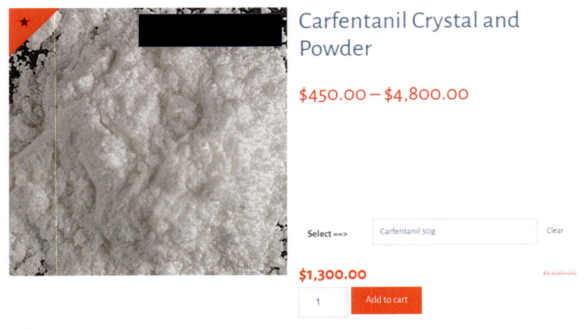

SOURCE: Vendor 3.
NOTE: We have redacted individual vendor and seller names and contact information.

Figure 4.5
Product Listing for Fentanyl Powder

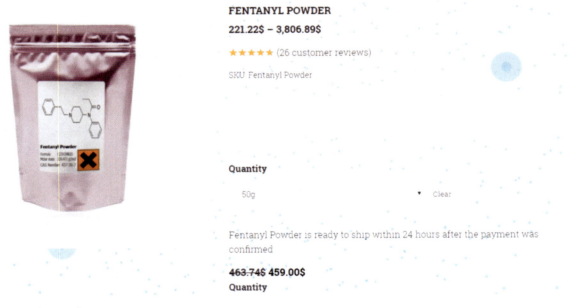

SOURCE: Vendor 4.
NOTE: The quantity offered in the dropdown menu ranged from 10 to 1,000 g.

OR distribut*) AND indict* AND headline (fentanyl). This resulted in 143 news items related to fentanyl distribution or trafficking. Not all of these press releases were related to different people, and not all were related to indictments—some pertained to arrests, convictions, or sentencing. The goal here was to ascertain the location of fentanyl distribution or trafficking and the accused's potential links to foreign fentanyl suppliers.

With the extracted series of press releases, we focused on unique cases related to fentanyl distribution and trafficking in Ohio and New England (Connecticut, Maine, Massachusetts, New Hampshire, Rhode Island, and Vermont). Of the press releases, 59 were reported to come from cases taking place or linked to Ohio or New England. We tasked a research assistant to read through these 59 press releases and tally the incidents in which the accused had explicit ties to a Chinese, Mexican, or Dominican source of fentanyl. Table 4.5 reports these tallies, showing that four of the 31 in Ohio were related to Chinese sources and that nine of the 28 in New England involved Mexican or Dominican trafficking sources. No press releases about New England mentioned China as a possible source, and none in Ohio mentioned anyone with a link to any Dominican or Mexican criminal organization. We were unable to infer the source of fentanyl or related substances for other distribution or trafficking events, although most of these involved people involved with domestic distribution close to retail.

This is not an analysis of federal legal action but of DOJ press releases we could capture in federal news. It does not cover state or local indictments, and it does not include additional data that might be found in federal indictments. Our research here can glean only data mentioned in these short releases, not full court documents and references to evidence supporting or denying the links with foreign suppliers. Nonetheless, this cursory examination of supply sources reported in federal legal actions align with what is seen in NFLIS data, suggesting that the supply of fentanyl in markets in New England might be dominated by traditional drug trafficking organizations with links to Mexico, whereas Ohio might be supplied to a greater extent by buyers importing product from China via the mail.

Summary

Understanding the delivery mechanisms and supply channels used to traffic fentanyl and related substances is an important law enforcement goal to help find better mechanisms or tools to detect these drugs. That said, the production of highly potent synthetic opioids introduces considerable challenges to drug interdiction. Unlike traditional drug threats, synthetic

Table 4.5
Federal Press Releases About Fentanyl Distribution or Trafficking in Ohio and New England, 2017–2018

Location	All Press Releases	Those Related to China	Those Related to Mexico or the Dominican Republic
Ohio	31	4	0
New England	28	0	9

SOURCE: Federal News Service press releases from between January 2017 and December 2018 in Ohio, Connecticut, Maine, Massachusetts, New Hampshire, Rhode Island, and Vermont.

opioids are produced by not only a handful of criminal groups but possibly scores of small- to medium-sized and independent laboratories (O'Connor, 2017); their potency-to-weight ratios make them profitable enough to ship tens of grams via the international postal system; and their availability via online vendors allows just about anyone to acquire these substances from the comfort of their own homes.

Research into the smuggling and distribution of synthetic opioids differs from that into traditional drug threats. Online vendors openly sell and ship product to buyers anywhere in the world, using legitimate postal and parcel services. There are many unknown dimensions to this evolving phenomenon. We attempted to validate findings using data from indictments and federal news releases. However, additional research is needed so that we can better understand the distribution of synthetic opioids.

However, the supply chain of these substances appears to be different from those for heroin or cocaine in that fentanyl can be mailed direct to buyers who make purchases online. Analysis here provides further insights into some of the mechanisms that online vendors, which claim to employ methods to circumvent customs, use.

First, vendors report regularly using the postal or other private consignment couriers to transmit packages to customers. They generally ship orders no larger than 1 kg. Larger amounts are offered upon request, but those might originate from domestic warehouses near customers. Second, the mention that many online vendors make of holding inventory in Europe, the United States, and elsewhere to avoid detection suggests that suppliers understand the risks and take steps to reduce it. At this time, there is no way to know what share of inventory is warehoused outside of China. However, knowing that inventory arrives in the United States via bulk container and cargo shipments might necessitate a recalibration of law enforcement strategy. Instead of targeting individual parcels arriving at mail facilities, law enforcement might consider prioritizing detection of bulk items that might conceal product destined for domestic warehouses. The recent seizure of 50 kg of nearly pure 4-fluoroisobutyryl fentanyl in Philadelphia is perhaps one example of a vendor's attempt to move inventory for warehousing in the United States.

Third, vendors are confident that their packages often slip by customs undetected and will reship product at no cost should a package get lost, stolen, or interdicted. Vendors understand customs and detection risks, preferring to ship via EMS (the international postal system). The Zheng organization noted the success rate of sending packages through the customs facility in New York. One online vendor noted the higher risk of sending product to Scandinavia. This might be an important data point, and U.S. law enforcement should enhance collaboration with counterparts in Norway, Sweden, Finland, and Denmark to better understand what detection methods or risk assessment tools are deployed in those countries.

If vendors are to be believed and their rates of success in shipping product to buyers in the United States are almost always successful, customs is seizing perhaps only a small proportion of total shipments. The alternative explanation is that online vendors have a high tolerance to loss given the low risk of arrest and prosecution and thus are claiming high rates of circumvention to entice prospective customers with false assurances. Given that the supply of these substances is unconventional, with vendors openly discussing their product and exclusive use of the postal system, law enforcement should start to think more creatively—if it has not already done so—to obtain additional information about packages. Engaging with online vendors and initiating controlled deliveries of smaller packages from China will provide additional data on the techniques used to avoid detection at IMFs. Likewise, if bulk shipments of product originate from warehouses in the United States, law enforcement and postal inspectors might be able to initiate controlled deliveries, working backward to identify the locations and operators of warehouses. Unlike traditional drug trafficking organizations, which employ criminal networks, overseas suppliers must rely almost entirely on the postal system for distribution purposes. In some ways, this presents an advantage for data collection and intelligence gathering because packages are tracked.

CHAPTER FIVE

Chemicals Associated with Cutting and Packaging Synthetic Opioids for Retail

Understanding the composition of drugs sold in retail might give law enforcement a picture of distribution trends and supply chains. Fentanyl and NSOs can be pressed with bulking agents into counterfeit prescription tablets or mixed with and sold as heroin. The lethal dose of fentanyl for an opioid-naïve person[1] is approximately 2 mg (European Monitoring Centre for Drugs and Drug Addiction [EMCDDA], 2015), equivalent to roughly two grains of salt. Ingesting drugs in such small quantities necessitates that these substances be mixed with other agents. Therefore, mapping the use of adulterants and diluents could help provide a more complete picture of supply trends (Dams et al., 2001). This might be particularly true for counterfeit tablets that contain fentanyl or another NSO.

However, the utility of such findings to CBP or other law enforcement agencies tasked with interdicting product before it arrives in the United States depends on where in the supply chain cutting agents are added. For example, if domestic dealers near drug markets obtain nearly pure synthetic opioids from vendors overseas and dilute them with inactive agents at home, understanding the chemicals associated with cutting such retail packages is of little use to CBP, which is tasked with detecting and interdicting packages arriving at POEs.

To gain insight into the variation of cutting agents, we used publicly available data, as well as information drawn from the analysis of scrapes of marketplaces and analyses of online vendor websites. Analysis of unclassified fentanyl signature analyses from DEA provides some limited insights into the chemical composition of seizures containing fentanyl and NSOs.

In response to a request from DHS S&T sponsors after initial discussions, this chapter first describes the terminology relevant to bulking or cutting agents used to increase the weight or alter the pharmacological effects of a drug sold in illicit retail markets. It then discusses the methodology and some findings from the analysis of HSOAC supplemental data regarding the supply of synthetic opioids from overseas.

Terminology

A standardized set of terms should aid in data collection, analysis, and reporting of drug seizures throughout the various chains of supply. By adopting standard terminology, federal authorities can better streamline data collection and reporting systems to allow for interagency data comparisons. This short section should be thought of as an initial step toward that end. A

---

[1] Someone without a tolerance to opioids, like a regular opioid user or pain patient would have.

more robust set of terms that captures the emergence of new components and a broader understanding of this problem can be better achieved through interagency coordination.

The lexicon presented here provides a glossary of terms that authorities can use to better describe the emerging trends and dimensions of adulterants and diluents found in seizures containing fentanyl and other NSOs. For various reasons, we exclude the use of street or slang terms for these drugs and focus on the technical components or elements that are used to describe them.

In building this lexicon of terms, we drew from two authoritative sources: the World Health Organization (WHO) and the EMCDDA. Table 5.1 lists many of these terms, some of which are used interchangeably. What is important to note is the difference between bulking and cutting agents: The latter might or might not be pharmacologically active or be designed to enhance the pharmacological effects of the drug in question. In contrast, bulking agents are merely intended to increase the weight of a retail drug product without changing its pharmacological effect. For example, non-psychoactive bulking agents, such as sucrose and lactose,

Table 5.1
Lexicon

Term	Definition
active pharmaceutical ingredient	The substance in a drug product that is biologically active
adulterant	Often synonymous with *cutting agent*. A substance added to a drug to increase its weight. It can be inert or pharmacologically active. It can be found in illicit powders, as well as tablets. Generally added near retail markets to enhance or mimic psychopharmacological effect.
bulking agent	See *excipient*.
cutting agent	Often synonymous with *adulterant*. A substance added to a drug to increase its weight. It can be inert or pharmacologically active. Generally added near retail markets to increase the weight of retail product and sometimes enhance or mimic psychopharmacological effect.
designer drug	A novel chemical substance with psychoactive properties, synthesized specifically to circumvent regulations on controlled substances. In response, these regulations now commonly cover novel substances and possible analogs of existing psychoactive substances. See *new psychoactive substance*.
diluent	See *excipient*.
excipient	An inactive substance that serves as the vehicle or medium for a drug or other active substance, often to increase the weight without changing the biological effects
filler	See *excipient*.
legal high	See *new psychoactive substance*.
new psychoactive substance	Sometimes synonymous with *designer drug* or *legal high*. Generally defined as a new narcotic or psychotropic drug, in pure form or in preparation, that is not controlled by the United Nations drug conventions or national laws but that might pose a public health threat comparable to that posed by substances listed in international conventions.
potentiating agent	An active substance that, often synergistically, increases or enhances the pharmacologic action of another drug
tablet binder	See *excipient*.

SOURCES: WHO, undated; EMCDDA, 2013.

are diluents and can be used to increase the weight of a drug product sold in retail. However, cutting agents, such as caffeine or lidocaine (which are psychoactive), are adulterants and can be used to enhance or alter the pharmacological effect of a drug while also increasing its gross weight.

Methodology

Understanding the composition of drug seizures, especially those at retail, would be best achieved by examining individual drug seizure data. This is particularly true of data on drug seizures at or near retail markets. Doing so would allow researchers to examine the chemical composition of drug seizures, including cutting agents, as well as the distribution of purity of seizures. Ideally, having domestic drug seizure data from DEA through the System to Retrieve Information from Drug Evidence (STRIDE) and its replacement, STARLiMS, would provide even more insights. However, these data were not available at the time of our analyses, so we used publicly available data from federal law enforcement and unclassified reports to understand the dimensions of this task. Further, we drew on our supplemental data analysis from scraped web data and qualitative evaluations of online vendors. We also included details from publicly available drug seizure data reported by law enforcement.

Limitations

Drug seizure data are not random samples of the population of retail drug transactions. Furthermore, we have insights into only those products that are seized, not the entire population of drugs—in this case, synthetic opioids. For example, CBP seizures of fentanyl at the southwest border are reportedly of very low purity, suggesting that they are made up largely of substances other than fentanyl, such as bulking agents, which are used to increase volume because fentanyl's potency requires dosing in minute amounts (perhaps 1 to 10 mg per tablet). These bulk, low-purity seizures are harder to conceal and thus have a higher probability of detection by law enforcement. In contrast, the high-purity, smaller shipments might escape detection, given that they are easier to conceal. This limitation is important to keep in mind when interpreting these findings.

Likewise, analyzing product descriptions of scraped marketplace data is limited to a single point in time and, although we assumed the perspective of a potential buyer, the product descriptions analyzed might not fully reflect the total population of product that vendors from China and other countries offer.

Findings

From public data analyzed in earlier chapters, we see a difference in the purity of fentanyl seizures depending on POE. Product seized at or near the southwest border are reportedly of low purity, roughly 5 to 10 percent (DEA, 2018c; Owen, 2018). This suggests that the majority of those individual seizures contain ingredients other than fentanyl. News media on seizures mention the increased incidence of seizures of counterfeit prescription pills containing fentanyl at the southwest border (Davis, 2018; DEA, 2018c; Nevano, 2018; Riggins, 2018). In these cases, product is pressed into tablets with some filling agent and imported in retail or near-retail form. Because of the potency of fentanyl and other NSOs, such drugs are dosed in minute quantities, requiring a filling agent for the final product to mimic prescription tablets. This stands in contrast with the convention that wholesale drug shipments are trafficked at higher purity, reducing the risk of interdiction due to conveying product containing bulking agents.

On the other hand, product seized at mail and ECC facilities is reportedly of very high purity, 95 percent or greater (DEA, 2018c; Owen, 2018). This indicates that such product is uncut and might be destined for distributors prior to retail distribution. The fact that such differences in the purity of seizures coincide with locations of seizure indicates variation in supply sources. Products seized at the southwest border in tablet form are reported to be of low purity but perhaps ready for retail distribution. Yet product coming by mail is reportedly of high purity and perhaps unlikely to be destined for immediate retail distribution.

The analysis of online vendors and marketplace listings suggests that the majority of product on offer from retailers overseas is highly pure. This coincides with CBP seizure analyses described in annual reports. We have no means of verification, but online retailers regularly report that their product is very pure. Some state percentages of "99%" or "99.9%" pure. If those claims are true, these products are unlikely to contain diluents or other added bulking agents.

Our analysis of scraped product descriptions indicates that the majority of items sold in marketplaces are of powder formulation. This finding might support law enforcement reports that high-purity product seized in mail facilities are generally high-purity powders.

When looking at DEA reports of NFLIS seizures reproduced in Table 3.2 in Chapter Three, we see that two-thirds of analyzed fentanyl cases contain no other drugs. However, about a quarter of fentanyl seizures in recent years also contained heroin, followed by other opioids at 4 percent. This, along with the fact that fentanyl is often offered as heroin or prescription opioids, is a notable insight. Analyses of heroin seizures in recent years could provide further understanding into cutting agents used in retail of fentanyl products. If dealers in the United States are replacing heroin with fentanyl to reduce costs, they might be using the same or similar bulking and cutting agents.

In recent years, DEA has assessed fentanyl seizures submitted to its laboratories in the United States. The FSPP analyzes seizures of drugs containing fentanyl. DEA notes that these results are not intended to "reflect U.S. market share, but rather a snapshot of samples" submitted to the seven DEA laboratories in a given year. Although these are not representative, chemical analysis sheds some additional light on the various diluents found in seizures, as well as the amount or purity of fentanyl in any given seizure.

We received publicly available FSPP reports covering the entire 2017 and 2018 calendar years. In both years, the majority of samples were submitted to either the New York or San Diego DEA regional laboratory. California and New York made up about half the weight of fentanyl seized in these reports. The FSPP improved its analytical methods in 2018 to permit better identification of fentanyl synthesis methods (i.e., Janssen or Siegfried).[2] Reports do not

---

[2] The chemical synthesis literature indicates that the Janssen method is more complex and requires more-specialized skills and a controlled environment to synthesize fentanyl. In contrast, the Siegfried method is generally considered an easier and less dangerous synthesis route (Yadav et al., 2010) and therefore possibly more attractive to clandestine operators.

indicate where in the supply chain those seizures were made (e.g., at retail or at wholesale). That said, the majority of exhibits analyzed were of powders, with most being wholesale amounts (defined as 1 kg or more). The FSPP did not include "seizures of very high purity fentanyl suspected as direct imports from China." We interpret this to mean that items seized at IMFs or ECC POEs were not included in the analysis. It is unclear what portion of seizures analyzed might arrive from Mexico or China (or theoretically produced domestically, for that matter).

The number of seizures analyzed decreased from 941 total exhibits in 2017 to 732 total exhibits in 2018. Between 2017 and 2018, the purity of fentanyl powder seized has increased in seizures larger than 10 g. The fentanyl content in wholesale powder seizures (e.g., those larger than 1 kg) increased from 6.6 percent ($n = 332$) to 7.8 percent ($n = 222$), on average.

In Table 5.2, we report the breakdown of exhibits (separated by powder and tablet) analyzed in the FSPP for 2017 and 2018. The table separates out fentanyl-related exhibits (i.e., analogs and other NSOs), focusing mostly on seizures containing fentanyl. Most seizure exhibits analyzed were of powder. The average purity did not appreciably change from 2017 to 2018, remaining steady at just more than 5 percent. Likewise, powder fentanyl exhibits ranged in purity from very little (0.1 percent) to almost pure (around 97 percent).

About three in ten exhibits also contained heroin in either year, aligning with publicly produced reports of NFLIS data. Of those that contained heroin, the purity of heroin and fentanyl declined, with the share of fentanyl declining more than the share of heroin has (from 4.8 percent to 2.9 percent for fentanyl, compared with 16.4 percent to 13 percent for heroin).

Table 5.2
Breakdown of Fentanyl Seizures Reported in the FSPP, 2017 and 2018

Characteristic	Powders		Tablets	
	2017	2018	2017	2018
Exhibits	692	568	72	100
Fentanyl-related exhibits	143	45	27	13
Weight, in kilograms	1,177	723	23	112
Fentanyl content	5.3%	5.2%	1.3 mg	1.5 mg
Range of fentanyl content	0.1–97.8%	0.1–96.8%	0.01–5.51 mg	0.02–4.84 mg
Percentage of seizures containing heroin	30	32	—	—
Diluents	Lactose (55%); mannitol (16%); inositol (9%); dipyrone (4%); other (16%)	Lactose (54%); mannitol (20%); inositol (12%); other (14%)	—	—
Synthesis method	Janssen (7%), remainder unknown	Janssen (94%, $n = 80$); Siegfried (6%, $n = 5$)	—	Janssen (14%), remainder unknown

SOURCES: DEA, 2018a, 2019.

NOTE: A small number of exhibits analyzed were neither tablet nor powder: eight liquid exhibits in 2017 and four tar exhibits in 2018.

In terms of diluents found in powder exhibits, more than half contained lactose. According to the fentanyl signature reports, about a sixth of powder exhibits in 2017 and a fifth in 2018 contained mannitol. This was followed by inositol and other diluents found in decreasing amounts.

In 2018, when the FSPP improved its analytical methods for synthesis determination, a majority of powder samples (94 percent, $n = 85$) tested were reportedly manufactured using the Janssen method.[3] The amount of fentanyl in tablet exhibits increased slightly between 2017 and 2018, from 1.3 mg to 1.5 mg. Lastly, in 2018, fewer exhibits analyzed contained fentanyl-related substances. In 2017, 19 percent of exhibits were for fentanyl-related substances, compared with just more than 8 percent in 2018.

Data from the FSPP suggest that the majority of seizures analyzed were of wholesale amounts (those larger than 1 kg), which might not indicate the true scope of adulteration or dilution of fentanyl-containing products sold in illicit markets. Furthermore, the FSPP did not indicate the diluents used in counterfeit tablets containing fentanyl or fentanyl-related substances. An analysis of heroin seizures might provide some additional information on common diluents or adulterants found in retail markets.

In the most-recent analyses we could find of domestic heroin seizures in the United States published in the literature, Coomber showed that three-quarters of the seizures ($n = 818$) contained several diluents and adulterants, including mannitol (39 percent), lactose (33 percent), starch (25 percent), quinine (23 percent), procaine (14 percent), diphenhydramine or caffeine (12 percent), paracetamol (10 percent), and dextrose (4 percent) (Coomber, 1999). However, the article notes that analysis did not permit determining purity of these cutting agents. Furthermore, the findings here are almost 25 years old, and dealers might have adopted use of other bulking or cutting agents. In a more recent analysis of heroin ($n = 325$) and synthetic opioid ($n = 156$) seizures from Kentucky and Vermont, authors found slight variation in cutting agents across the two sets of drugs and that caffeine and quinine or quinidine were most-common adulterants. Seizures of synthetic opioids, such as fentanyl, reported greater frequency of adulteration with diphenhydramine, acetaminophen, benzocaine, xylazine, and diltiazem (Fiorentin et al., 2018). We reproduce the relevant sections of their analysis in Table 5.3.

Summary

The analysis of online vendors and marketplace listings suggests that the majority of product on offer from retailers overseas is highly pure. This coincides with CBP seizure analyses described in annual reports. We have no means of verification, but online retailers regularly report that their product is very pure. Some state percentages of "99%" or "99.9%" pure. If true, these products are unlikely to contain diluents or other added bulking agents.

---

[3] It is not clear what portion of the total number of exhibits were analyzed using this method to determine synthesis route because only 85 samples (of a total of 732 seizure exhibits) were reportedly analyzed in the 2018 FSPP. At this time, we are not aware of any unclassified reports to indicate which production source (either Mexican drug traffickers or Chinese laboratories) prefers which synthesis method. However, the chemical synthesis literature has documented that the Janssen method is more complex and requires more-specialized skills and a controlled environment to synthesize fentanyl. In contrast, the Siegfried method is generally considered an easier and less dangerous synthesis route (Yadav et al., 2010) and therefore possibly more attractive to clandestine operators.

Table 5.3
Percentage of Common Adulterants in Heroin and Synthetic Opioid Seizures in Kentucky and Vermont in 2018

Adulterant	Heroin (n = 325)	Fentanyl (n = 109)	Furanyl Fentanyl (n = 16)	Acetyl Fentanyl (n = 16)	Butyryl Fentanyl (n = 1)	U-4 (n = 4)
Levamisole	4.3	9.2	—	—	—	25.0
Phenacetin	5.2	2.8	18.8	6.3	—	—
Quinine or quinidine	42.5	47.7	31.3	43.8	—	25.0
Caffeine	51.1	45.9	25.0	25.0	—	75.0
Acetaminophen	6.5	13.8	—	6.3	—	25.0
Procaine	22.2	22.9	6.3	6.3	—	—
Lidocaine	17.2	17.4	25.0	50.0	—	—
Diphenhydramine	6.8	26.6	12.5	18.8	—	—
Diltiazem	7.4	15.6	—	—	—	—
Benzocaine	0.6	1.8	—	—	—	—
Xylazine	4.6	11.0	—	—	—	—
Dipyrone	1.2	3.7	—	—	—	—
Aminopyrine	3.7	11.0	—	—	—	—
Hydroxyzine	0.3	—	—	—	—	—

SOURCE: Fiorentin et al., 2018.

Our analysis of scraped product descriptions indicates that that the majority of items sold in marketplaces are of powder formulation. This finding could support law enforcement reports that high-purity product is seized in mail facilities.

When looking at DEA reports of NFLIS seizures reproduced in Table 3.5 in Chapter Three, we see that two-thirds of analyzed fentanyl cases contain no other drug mixtures. However, about a quarter of fentanyl seizures in recent years also contain heroin, followed by other opioids at 4 percent. This, along with the fact that fentanyl is often offered as heroin or prescription opioids, is a notable insight. Analysis of heroin seizures in recent years could provide further understanding into cutting agents used in retail of fentanyl products. If dealers in the United States are replacing heroin with fentanyl to reduce costs, they might be using the same or similar bulking and cutting agents.

Unclassified fentanyl signature reports show that adulteration and dilution do occur, with lactose and mannitol the most-common diluents. The fentanyl content analyzed in these reports is steady over two years. However, without knowing where exactly these seizures occurred, determining their source of origin is difficult. DEA notes that it is improving its synthesis determination methods but that, in 2018, the majority of seizures analyzed (85) were manufactured using the Janssen synthesis method. This suggests a higher degree of synthesis knowledge and available resources.

CHAPTER SIX

Conclusions and Recommendations

The opioid overdose crisis has continued to accelerate thanks to the arrival of potent synthetic opioids, such as fentanyl and related substances. Although several synthetic opioids have legitimate medical applications, the majority of overdoses are due to illicitly manufactured imports. To support drug interdiction efforts at U.S. POEs, we evaluated publicly available data to better understand the dimensions of the consumption and supply of these substances. To provide insights into this new and quickly evolving phenomenon, we summarize in this chapter our key conclusions for each of the four tasks undertaken. We also offer recommendations for DHS and CBP to consider.

Conclusions

The Number of Deaths from Overdose of Synthetic Opioids Has Trended Upward over Time

According to a descriptive analysis of overdose mortality data for recent years, national trends indicate that synthetic opioid deaths are on the rise and reaching alarmingly high levels in some states (and especially in some counties) across various drug classes. In 2013, nationally, the synthetic opioid overdose rate was one per 100,000 population; by 2017, this had jumped to nine per 100,000 population, surpassing heroin and prescription opioid overdoses by a factor of 2. In 2017, the ten states with the highest per capita drug overdose death rates involving synthetic opioids were, in descending order, West Virginia, Ohio, New Hampshire, Maryland, Massachusetts, Maine, Connecticut, Rhode Island, Delaware, and Kentucky.

States vary in drug overdose death rates involving synthetic opioids. Furthermore, within states, there is variation at the county level. To identify those counties with high rates, we used a threshold rate of 20 synthetic opioid overdose deaths per 100,000 population to compare county rates within and across states. As a point of reference, the national rate of synthetic opioid deaths was 6.2 per 100,000 population in 2016 and nine per 100,000 population in 2017. Our cutoff was two to three times higher than these national rates. Within the states with the highest 2017 synthetic opioid death rates, the county-level results, which suggest that this problem is localized, are informative about the variation occurring within states.

The county-level trends in synthetic opioid deaths can help inform CBP's understanding of ways to improve its targeting of parcels, whether shipped by mail or by private courier, that might contain synthetic opioids. An examination of overdose deaths at the ZIP Code level could provide some additional information to help law enforcement screen inbound packages that arrive at mail facilities. Although the ZIP Codes for the counties where the decedents in synthetic opioid fatalities had resided might not be perfect proxies for where incoming packages are addressed, county hot spots and associated ZIP Codes could be a first-level proxy for destinations of imported drug shipments. When juxtaposing these overdose death data alongside NFLIS counts, we can get a sense of which areas are likely to be supplied by synthetic opioids that arrive by mail versus those that arrive via traditional drug trafficking routes that cross land borders.

Trends in Synthetic Opioid Seizures Are Evolving

Our analyses of publicly available data indicate that the number of seizures containing fentanyl and related substances is increasing over time. In addition, the growing variation of fentanyl analogs reported in NFLIS suggests an evolution in synthesis and manufacturing. Many of the new analogs reported in NFLIS data have never been reported in drug markets until now.

Both the rising number of fentanyl-related exhibits and the variation in chemicals could be contributing to harms (such as overdoses) that drug users experience. The diffusion of fentanyl increases the risk that street-sourced drugs are tainted with potent opioids. Additionally, users (and perhaps dealers) might not be aware of the morphine-equivalent of many fentanyl analogs.

Across the United States, the supply of illicitly manufactured synthetic opioids varies. Several regions report high per capita rates of seizures that contain fentanyl and related chemicals. The East North Central and New England census divisions, which encompass parts of Appalachia, report the highest per capita rates. The upward trend in NFLIS reports is positively correlated with trends in overdose death rates for synthetic opioids summarized above.

NFLIS data further indicate considerable geographic variation in the types of chemicals present. In states in New England, fentanyl predominates in NFLIS observations. In contrast, some states, such as Ohio and some in the Middle Atlantic, report greater variation in the types of chemicals reported, including counts for super-potent opioids, such as carfentanil. For example, about 45 percent of counts for Ohio in 2017 were fentanyl analogs. The distinction in the types of chemicals that laboratories in different states reported suggests that these markets might be supplied by different sources. In the case of markets in New England, the lack of variation in chemicals suggests fewer suppliers or entrants to the market. In these cases, markets might be supplied by Mexican traffickers. States that report greater variation in seizure data might be supplied by online vendors from China that offer a multitude of ever-changing analogs. A preliminary examination of federal news releases for arrests and indictments supports this hypothesis.

However, there are several limitations to our analysis of the NFLIS data. Without having individual-level seizure observations, we cannot determine the total amount of fentanyl and fentanyl-related substances seized in the United States. DEA data indicate that about 70 percent of seizures containing fentanyl are fentanyl only (i.e., absent any other drug). Only about a quarter of fentanyl-related seizures contain heroin. Without knowing whether seizures are of product at the wholesale level or retail level, we are unable to determine where in the supply chain the mixing is occurring. Our analysis suggests variation in supply sources, with chemicals from China concentrated in some states but perhaps not in others. Understanding the variation on the ground in these different sources of supply could help improve law enforcement's response.

The Supply and Trafficking of Synthetic Opioids Differ from Those for Other Drugs

The production of highly potent synthetic opioids introduces considerable challenges to drug interdiction. Unlike traditional drug threats, synthetic opioids are not produced by a handful of criminal groups but by possibly scores of small- to medium-sized independent laboratories; their potency-to-weight ratio make them profitable enough to ship tens of grams via the international postal system; and their availability via online vendors allows just about anyone to acquire these substances from the comfort of their own homes.

The supply chain of these substances is also novel. Unlike heroin or cocaine, which must be clandestinely produced and smuggled across borders, synthetic opioids can be produced in underregulated laboratories and shipped through legitimate supply networks, such as the postal system. We show that vendors in Asia regularly use the postal or other private consignment couriers to transmit packages to customers and generally ship orders no larger than 1 kg. Larger amounts are offered upon request, but those might originate from domestic warehouses near customers. The discussion among many online vendors of holding inventory in Europe, the United States, and elsewhere as a means to avoid detection suggests that suppliers understand the risk of detection and are taking steps to reduce it. Currently, there is no way to know what share of inventory is warehoused outside of China; however, knowing that inventory arrives in the United States via bulk container and cargo shipments could allow further recalibration of law enforcement's strategy. For example, instead of targeting individual parcels arriving at mail facilities, law enforcement might consider prioritizing detection of bulk items that might conceal product destined for domestic warehouses. The recent seizure of 50 kg of nearly pure 4-fluoroisobutyryl fentanyl at the Philadelphia POE might be one example of a vendor's attempt to move inventory for warehousing in the United States.

Vendors appear to understand customs and detection risks, preferring to ship via the international postal system. Furthermore, vendors often assess the risk of interdiction as being low and even offer to reship an order at no cost should a package be lost, stolen, or interdicted. If vendors are to be believed and their rates of success in shipping product to buyers in the United States are almost always successful, customs is perhaps seizing only a small proportion of total shipments. Given that the supply of these substances is unconventional, with vendors openly discussing their product and use of the postal system, law enforcement might want to think more creatively—if it has not already done so—about how to obtain additional information about packages. As discussed in the "Recommendations" section, engaging with online vendors and initiating controlled deliveries of smaller packages from China is one way to obtain additional data on the techniques used to avoid detection at IMFs.

Additional Information Is Needed on the Chemicals Associated with Cutting and Packaging of Synthetic Opioids for Retail

To gain insight into the variation of cutting agents, we used publicly available and unclassified data, as well as information drawn from analysis of web scrapes of marketplaces and of online vendors' websites. Our analysis of online vendors and marketplace listings suggests that the majority of product on offer from retailers overseas is highly pure. This is consistent with CBP seizure analyses described in annual reports. A review of online vendors' product descriptions indicates that a majority of items sold in the marketplaces are of powder formulation. This finding supports law enforcement reports of high-purity powder being seized in mail facilities.

NFLIS reports of seizures indicate that two-thirds of analyzed fentanyl cases contain no other drug mixtures. However, about a quarter of fentanyl seizures in recent years also contain heroin, followed by other opioids at 4 percent. Fentanyl signature profiling reports also show a similar share of fentanyl seizures containing heroin and that the purity of fentanyl seizures has remained constant in recent years. This, along with the fact that fentanyl is often offered as heroin or prescription opioids, is a notable insight. Analysis of heroin seizures in recent years could provide further understanding into the cutting agents used in retail of fentanyl products. If dealers in the United States are replacing heroin with fentanyl to reduce costs, they might be using the same or similar bulking and cutting agents. Without assessing individual seizure data, however, we were limited in our ability to understand the cutting and bulking agents included in the retail distribution of fentanyl and NSOs.

Recommendations

Use Mortality and Morbidity Data to Inform Targeting of Packages from Abroad

Understanding the levels and trends of synthetic opioid mortality data reflect only the tip of the iceberg, given the large number of nonfatal drug overdoses in addition to those that result in death. Nonetheless, these data might be used to help CBP (as well as USPIS) target packages from abroad that are destined for markets where synthetic opioids pose the greatest threat.

We recognize that state and county hot spots where synthetic opioid deaths are occurring (i.e., reflecting consumption or exposure) might not be perfect proxies for where imported drug shipments are arriving and that understanding where synthetic opioids are used, as proxied by state- and county-specific overdose death figures, might not exactly correspond to supply. It is also possible, as noted by the warehousing phenomenon reported by vendors, that dealers are outside areas of high rates of use. Thus, the targeting information presented here might fail to truly represent the risk presented by individual parcels.

As for the use of synthetic opioids, federal law enforcement might want to consider targeting detection resources, such as canine units trained in detection of synthetic opioids or infrared spectroscopy equipment, and screening efforts at items addressed to final destinations in ZIP Codes where fatal synthetic opioid overdoses are occurring. This is especially true in states that report to NFLIS higher shares of fentanyl-related substances, which are likely to arrive by mail. Comparing county-level overdose deaths and county- or sub-state-level NFLIS data could help to improve targeting.

Improve Data Collection and Analysis of Drug Seizures

To improve data collection and analysis, drug seizure data collection at POEs should be recorded across all IMFs and ECCs, as well as POEs on the border, and inputted into a central standardized data repository. Including additional measures on each seizure, such as purity, concealment methods, and analysis of other chemicals that might be present (e.g., diluents, adulterants, impurities), will also help improve analysis to enhance targeting. Although these increase costs to agencies, it is important to collect as much information as possible on a fast-moving problem, especially given how little data are currently available.

Collecting reliable and comparable data across facilities will help increase the sample of drug interdiction observations, improving metrics and threat analytics, which can better inform interdiction strategies. The lack of standardized data input and collection complicates analyses. We recommend that relevant DHS components make considerable efforts to standardize and streamline data collection so that field operations do not have to manually input values but rather can select items from a predetermined set of options. Doing so will allow generation of automated reports, letting law enforcement quickly assess trends across and within POEs.

Enhance Cooperation with Other Federal Agencies and Departments to Better Understand the Supply of Synthetic Opioids

We recommend that CBP enhance cooperation with other relevant departments and agencies across the federal government to better understand the dimensions of the supply of fentanyl and NSOs. Given the significant challenges presented by this new drug threat, an interagency working group that meets regularly and reduces barriers to information sharing will help improve law enforcement's understanding of this problem.

For example, the seizure of counterfeit pills at the border suggests that supply chains are evolving in unexpected ways. Traditionally, Mexican drug traffickers would smuggle higher-purity product in uncut forms. Diluting or adulterating would generally occur closer to retail. Smuggling smaller but higher-purity content makes sense from a risk-mitigation standpoint. Nevertheless, the smuggling of relatively impure but full-strength pressed counterfeit pills ready for retail over the border defies this traditional logic. Perhaps Mexican cartels feel that the risk of detection of pill pressing is lower in Mexico or that they can better ensure product quality and consistency or more readily produce on industrial scale south of the border given lower costs of labor. Regardless of the reason, CBP needs to better understand the nature of fentanyl products in retail markets to inform interdiction strategies. This can be done only by using law enforcement data of retail markets or from intelligence gathered by law enforcement in the United States, such as DEA, and from sources in Mexico where pills are manufactured—data that CBP does not capture in its day-to-day operations.

Matching analytical samples of fentanyl seized at or near the southwest border with samples seized elsewhere can help improve signature analysis, especially as it pertains to the use of diluents in counterfeit tablets. DEA does currently map fentanyl signatures based on chemical analyses of impurities through the FSPP, but there are only a handful of instances of successful matches, and, until recently, DEA was unable to determine synthesis methods for most fentanyl seizures. Having a better analytical picture of synthesis methods, adulterants or diluents used, and purity figures can help improve our understanding of the various dimensions of the supply of synthetic opioids.

Compile and Compare Seizure Data with Counterparts in Law Enforcement and Customs Agencies in Other Countries

The fact that most of these chemicals are supplied via the international mail system could mean that law enforcement and customs in other countries are experiencing similar challenges and threats. Pooling seizure observations that arrive by mail or ECC will better inform current and future threats. We recommend that CBP reach out to counterpart law enforcement and border-protection services in North America and Europe to inquire about specific customs interdiction information and practices. For example, one online vendor noted that customs in Scandinavia were likelier than other European destinations to seize shipments. CBP should inquire with partners abroad to learn about innovative techniques but more importantly to pool global data on seizures. Increasing the number of observations of seizures from around the world could improve law enforcement's understanding of the delivery and supply methods of online vendors.

Conduct Controlled Deliveries for Analytic Purposes

Unlike traditional drug interdiction, the supply of fentanyl and NSOs is often advertised openly on the surface web. This presents law enforcement with a unique opportunity to gain a considerable amount of insight into the operations and strategies of online vendors overseas. Regularly conducting purchases from online vendors would allow law enforcement to understand how successful their detection methods are, as well as enhance detection metrics. Vendors regularly mention the high rate of success in circumventing customs. Conducting controlled deliveries at regular intervals would offer a window into how product escapes detection.

Also, law enforcement might want to consider initiating controlled deliveries of larger amounts, tracking orders back to the points of origin to locate warehouses. Vendors suggest that bulk orders (e.g., often larger than 1 kg) are available upon request. It is implied that such larger orders originate from domestic warehouses, rather than shipped internationally. Unlike criminal drug trafficking organizations, online vendors do not have supply networks and must rely almost exclusively on USPS and private couriers to move product. Although this is convenient for vendors, allowing them to tap into markets around the globe, it can also be a weakness. Relying on legitimate supply routes allows law enforcement to work backward to build cases.

Target Bulk Shipments from China at Points of Entry

Vendors regularly discuss warehousing product in the domestic United States. There has been at least one case of a facility warehousing product in Woburn, Massachusetts (see *Zheng*, 2018). If vendors are increasingly stockpiling product in the United States, CBP might be focusing its efforts on smaller and less important targets. Although CBP is making efforts by targeting individual packages arriving at mail and ECC facilities, there could be greater concern if vendors move to domestic warehousing. In effect, an order can be placed and fulfilled in a matter of days without ever crossing international boundaries. Vendors recognize the risks of detection at IMFs and ECC facilities and thus utilize domestic warehouses to avoid interdiction. As documented in DOJ indictments and recent bulk seizures, fentanyl and other NSOs arrive in the United States in bulk via cargo shipments. Targeting these larger shipments could have a greater impact on downstream markets.

References

Andersen, Travis, "Feds Nab Eight in Sprawling Drug Ring That Spanned from Mexico to Springfield," *Boston Globe*, March 22, 2018. As of March 21, 2019:
https://www.bostonglobe.com/metro/2018/03/22/
feds-nab-eight-sprawling-drug-ring-that-spanned-from-mexico-springfield/QVFj0xTPcWm33yFDMw1zkK/
story.html

Baum, Richard J., acting director, Office of National Drug Control Policy, Executive Office of the President, "Attachment: Response to Questions Concerning Fentanyl," letter to Greg Walden, chair of the U.S. House of Representatives Committee on Energy and Commerce; Tim Murphy, chair of the U.S. House of Representatives Committee on Energy and Commerce Subcommittee on Oversight and Investigations; Frank Pallone, Jr., ranking member, U.S. House of Representatives Committee on Energy and Commerce; and Diana DeGette, ranking member, U.S. House of Representatives Committee on Energy and Commerce Subcommittee on Oversight and Investigations, Washington, D.C., March 29, 2017. As of March 21, 2019:
https://archives-energycommerce.house.gov/sites/republicans.energycommerce.house.gov/files/
documents/20170329ONDCP_Response.pdf

CBP—*See* U.S. Customs and Border Protection.

CDC—*See* Centers for Disease Control and Prevention.

Centers for Disease Control and Prevention, "Multiple Cause of Death Data," last reviewed December 6, 2018a. As of March 22, 2019:
https://wonder.cdc.gov/mcd.html

———, "Synthetic Opioid Overdose Data," last updated December 19, 2018b. As of March 21, 2019:
https://www.cdc.gov/drugoverdose/data/fentanyl.html

China Post, "List of Charges for International Letters—Post Items," undated. As of March 22, 2019:
http://english.chinapost.com.cn/html1/category/1408/4048-1.htm

Ciccarone, Daniel, "Fentanyl in the US Heroin Supply: A Rapidly Changing Risk Environment," *International Journal of Drug Policy*, Vol. 46, August 2017, pp. 107–111.

Coomber, Ross, "The Cutting of Heroin in the United States in the 1990s," *Journal of Drug Issues*, Vol. 29, No. 1, 1999, pp. 17–35.

Dams, R., T. Benijts, W. E. Lambert, D. L. Massart, and A. P. De Leenheer, "Heroin Impurity Profiling: Trends Throughout a Decade of Experimenting," *Forensic Science International*, Vol. 123, Nos. 2–3, December 1, 2001, pp. 81–88.

Davis, Kristina, "20,000 Fentanyl Pills Seized at Border in San Diego, Beating Record Set Last Week," *San Diego Union-Tribune*, August 8, 2018. As of March 21, 2019:
https://www.sandiegouniontribune.com/news/courts/sd-me-fentanyl-seizure-20180808-story.html

DEA—*See* U.S. Drug Enforcement Administration.

EMCDDA—*See* European Monitoring Centre for Drugs and Drug Addiction.

European Monitoring Centre for Drugs and Drug Addiction, "Brief Glossary of Chemical and Biochemical Terms," last updated May 8, 2013. As of March 23, 2019:
http://www.emcdda.europa.eu/publications/drug-profiles/glossary

————, "Fentanyl Drug Profile," last updated January 8, 2015. As of March 23, 2019:
http://www.emcdda.europa.eu/publications/drug-profiles/fentanyl

Federal News Service, homepage, undated. As of March 23, 2019:
http://www.fednews.com/

Fiorentin, T. R., A. J. Krotulski, D. M. Martin, T. Browne, J. Triplett, T. Conti, and B. K. Logan, "Detection of Cutting Agents in Drug-Positive Seized Exhibits Within the United States," *Journal of Forensic Sciences*, November 28, 2018.

Gladden, R. Matthew, Pedro Martinez, and Puja Seth, "Fentanyl Law Enforcement Submissions and Increases in Synthetic Opioid–Involved Overdose Deaths: 27 States, 2013–2014," *Morbidity and Mortality Weekly Report*, Vol. 65, No. 33, August 26, 2016, pp. 837–843. As of March 24, 2019:
https://www.cdc.gov/mmwr/volumes/65/wr/mm6533a2.htm

Hedegaard, Holly, Margaret Warner, and Arialdi M. Miniño, *Drug Overdose Deaths in the United States, 1999–2016*, Hyattsville, Md.: Centers for Disease Control and Prevention, National Center for Health Statistics, Data Brief 294, December 2017. As of March 21, 2019:
https://www.cdc.gov/nchs/products/databriefs/db294.htm

Hernandez, Esteban L., "Feds Announce Largest Fentanyl Bust in Connecticut History," *New Haven Register*, May 19, 2016. As of March 21, 2019:
https://www.nhregister.com/connecticut/article/Feds-announce-largest-fentanyl-bust-in-11331593.php

Lamy, Francois, and Raminta Daniulaityte, *Collecting and Analyzing Cryptomarket Data on Novel Synthetic Opioids*, College Park, Md.: University of Maryland, Center for Substance Abuse Research, National Drug Early Warning System, October 24, 2018. As of March 21, 2019:
https://ndews.umd.edu/resources/collecting-and-analyzing-cryptomarket-data-novel-synthetic-opioids

Mars, Sarah G., Philippe Bourgois, George Karandinos, Fernando Montero, and Daniel Ciccarone, "The Textures of Heroin: User Perspectives on 'Black Tar' and Powder Heroin in Two US Cities," *Journal of Psychoactive Drugs*, Vol. 48, No. 4, September–October 2016, pp. 270–278.

Mars, S. G., D. Rosenblum, and D. Ciccarone, "Illicit Fentanyls in the Opioid Street Market: Desired or Imposed?" *Addiction*, December 4, 2018.

National Forensic Laboratory Information System, Diversion Control Division, Drug Enforcement Administration, U.S. Department of Justice, "National Forensic Laboratory Information System Questions and Answers (Q&A)," undated. As of March 23, 2019:
https://www.nflis.deadiversion.usdoj.gov/DesktopModules/ReportDownloads/Reports/2k17NFLISQA.pdf

————, *NHFLIS-DRUG 2017 Annual Report*, Springfield, Va., DEA PRB 09-12-18-39, September 2018. As of March 21, 2019:
https://www.nflis.deadiversion.usdoj.gov/DesktopModules/ReportDownloads/Reports/
NFLIS-Drug-AR2017.pdf

NFLIS—*See* National Forensic Laboratory Information System.

Nevano, Gregory C., "Homeland Security Investigations, Border Search Authority, and Investigative Approaches to Fentanyl Smuggling," *United States Attorneys' Bulletin*, Vol. 66, No. 4, July 2018, pp. 57–63. As of March 21, 2019:
https://www.justice.gov/usao/page/file/1083791/download

O'Connor, Sean, *Fentanyl: China's Deadly Export to the United States*, Washington, D.C.: U.S.–China Economic and Security Review Commission, staff research report, February 1, 2017. As of March 21, 2019:
https://www.uscc.gov/Research/fentanyl-china%E2%80%99s-deadly-export-united-states

Office of Inspector General, U.S. Postal Service, *Use of Postal Service Network to Facilitate Illicit Drug Distribution*, Arlington, Va., audit report SAT-AR-18-002, September 28, 2018. As of March 21, 2019:
https://www.uspsoig.gov/document/use-postal-service-network-facilitate-illicit-drug-distribution

Owen, Todd C., executive assistant commissioner, Office of Field Operations, U.S. Customs and Border Protection, U.S. Department of Homeland Security, "Combatting the Opioid Crisis: Exploiting Vulnerabilities in International Mail," testimony before the U.S. Senate Committee on Homeland Security and Governmental Affairs Permanent Subcommittee on Investigations, Washington, D.C., January 25, 2018. As of March 21, 2019:
https://www.hsgac.senate.gov/imo/media/doc/Owen%20Testimony.pdf

Pardo, Bryce, and Peter Reuter, "Facing Fentanyl: Should the USA Consider Trialling Prescription Heroin?" *Lancet Psychiatry*, Vol. 5, No. 8, August 1, 2018, pp. 613–615.

Perez, Robert E., acting executive assistant commissioner, Office of Operations Support, U.S. Customs and Border Protection, U.S. Department of Homeland Security, "Fentanyl and Fentanyl Analogues," testimony before the U.S. Sentencing Commission hearing, Washington, D.C., December 5, 2017. As of March 21, 2019:
https://www.ussc.gov/sites/default/files/pdf/amendment-process/public-hearings-and-meetings/20171205/Perez.pdf

Permanent Subcommittee on Investigations, Committee on Homeland Security and Governmental Affairs, U.S. Senate, *Combatting the Opioid Crisis: Exploiting Vulnerabilities in International Mail*, Washington, D.C., staff report, 2018. As of March 21, 2019:
https://www.hsgac.senate.gov/imo/media/doc/Combatting%20the%20Opioid%20Crisis%20-%20Exploiting%20Vulnerabilities%20in%20International%20Mail1.pdf

Public Law 107-210, Trade Act of 2002, August 6, 2002. As of March 22, 2019:
https://www.govinfo.gov/app/details/PLAW-107publ210

Public Law 115-271, Substance Use–Disorder Prevention That Promotes Opioid Recovery and Treatment (SUPPORT) for Patients and Communities Act, October 24, 2018.

Reuter, P., "Seizure of Drugs," in Jerome H. Jaffe, ed., *Encyclopedia of Drugs and Alcohol*, New York: MacMillan Library Reference USA, 1995.

Riggins, Alex, "Teen Charged in Largest-Ever Seizure of Fentanyl Pills at U.S. Border," *Los Angeles Times*, August 3, 2018. As of March 21, 2019:
https://www.latimes.com/local/lanow/la-me-fentanyl-seized-20180803-story.html

Ruhm, Christopher J., "Corrected US Opioid-Involved Drug Poisoning Deaths and Mortality Rates, 1999–2015," *Addiction*, Vol. 113, No. 7, July 2018, pp. 1339–1344.

Scholl, Lawrence, Puja Seth, Mbabazi Kariisa, Nana Wilson, and Grant Baldwin, "Drug and Opioid-Involved Overdose Deaths—United States, 2013–2017," *Morbidity and Mortality Weekly*, Vol. 67, No. 5152, January 4, 2019, pp. 1419–1427. As of July 11, 2019:
https://www.cdc.gov/mmwr/volumes/67/wr/mm675152e1.htm?s_cid=mm675152e1_w

Seth, Puja, Lawrence Scholl, Rose A. Rudd, and Sarah Bacon, "Overdose Deaths Involving Opioids, Cocaine, and Psychostimulants—United States, 2015–2016," *Morbidity and Mortality Weekly Report*, Vol. 67, No. 12, March 30, 2018, pp. 349–358. As of March 21, 2019:
http://dx.doi.org/10.15585/mmwr.mm6712a1

Townsend, Mark, "Dark Web Dealers Voluntarily Ban Deadly Fentanyl," *Guardian*, December 1, 2018. As of March 21, 2019:
https://www.theguardian.com/society/2018/dec/01/dark-web-dealers-voluntary-ban-deadly-fentanyl

United States of America v. Fujing Zheng, indictment, case 1:18-cr-00474-JRA, document 1, August 17, 2018. As of March 21, 2019:
https://www.justice.gov/opa/press-release/file/1089101/download

United States of America v. Jian Zhang, superseding indictment, case 3:17-cr-00206-DLH, document 50, January 18, 2018. As of March 23, 2019:
https://www.justice.gov/opa/press-release/file/1058216/download

U.S. Attorney's Office, District of Massachusetts, U.S. Department of Justice, "Lawrence Man and Dominican National Indicted for Fentanyl Conspiracy," press release, July 11, 2018a. As of March 21, 2019:
https://www.justice.gov/usao-ma/pr/lawrence-man-and-dominican-national-indicted-fentanyl-conspiracy

———, "Dominican National Indicted for Distributing Fentanyl and Heroin," press release, August 31, 2018b. As of March 21, 2019:
https://www.justice.gov/usao-ma/pr/dominican-national-indicted-distributing-fentanyl-and-heroin

U.S. Customs and Border Protection, "Philadelphia CBP Seizes Nearly $1.7 Million in Fentanyl Shipped from China," press release, June 28, 2018. As of March 21, 2019:
https://www.cbp.gov/newsroom/local-media-release/
philadelphia-cbp-seizes-nearly-17-million-fentanyl-shipped-china

U.S. Drug Enforcement Administration, U.S. Department of Justice, *2017 National Drug Threat Assessment*, DEA-DCT-040-17, October 2017. As of March 26, 2019:
https://www.dea.gov/sites/default/files/2018-07/DIR-040-17_2017-NDTA.pdf

———, *Fentanyl Signature Profiling Program*, 2018a.

———, "Schedules of Controlled Substances: Temporary Placement of Fentanyl-Related Substances in Schedule I," *Federal Register*, Vol. 83, No. 25, February 6, 2018b, pp. 5188–5192.

———, *2018 National Drug Threat Assessment*, DEA-DCT-DIR-032-18, October 2018c. As of March 21, 2019:
https://www.hsdl.org/?view&did=818528

———, *Fentanyl Signature Profiling Program*, January 2019.

Vardanyan, R. S., and V. J. Hruby, "Fentanyl-Related Compounds and Derivatives: Current Status and Future Prospects for Pharmaceutical Applications," *Future Medicinal Chemistry*, Vol. 6, No. 4, March 2014, pp. 385–412.

WHO—*See* World Health Organization.

WHOIS, homepage, undated. As of March 23, 2019:
https://whois.icann.org/en

Wish, Eric D., Amy Billing, Eleanor Erin Artigiani, Zachary Dezman, Bradford Schwartz, and Jordan Pueschel, *Drug Early Warning from Re-Testing Biological Samples: Maryland Hospital Study*, Washington, D.C.: Office of National Drug Control Policy, Executive Office of the President, July 2018. As of March 21, 2019:
https://umd.app.box.com/s/anskcsqajc7nk0wdegzrn4rupf4m61gb

World Health Organization, "Management of Substance Abuse: Lexicon of Alcohol and Drug Terms Published by the World Health Organization," undated. As of March 23, 2019:
https://www.who.int/substance_abuse/terminology/who_lexicon/en/

Xu, Jiaquan, Sherry L. Murphy, Kenneth D. Kochanek, Brigham Bastian, and Elizabeth Arias, "Deaths: Final Data for 2016," *National Vital Statistics Report*, Vol. 67, No. 5, July 26, 2018. As of July 11, 2019:
https://www.cdc.gov/nchs/data/nvsr/nvsr67/nvsr67_05.pdf

Yadav, Poonam, Jitendra S. Chauhan, K. Ganesan, Pradeep K. Gupta, Deepali Chauhan, and P. D. Gokulan, "Synthetic Methodology and Structure Activity Relationship Study of N-[1-(2-phenylethyl)-piperidin-4-yl]-propionamides," *Der Pharmacia Sinica*, Vol. 1, No. 3, 2010, pp. 126–139. As of March 21, 2019:
http://www.imedpub.com/abstract/synthetic-methodology-and-structure-activity-relationship-study-of-n12ph
enylethylpiperidin4ylpropionamides-16938.html